"Aguirre and Galen have raised the bar for self-help resources in the borderline personality disorder (BPD) community. Their wisdom and compassion shine through the lines of this text, creatively identifying common problems and effective solutions. For the person in recovery, they offer tools for problem solving to promote stability; and for therapists, and especially for professionals in training, they provide an opportunity to understand the individual experience of living with BPD—an accomplishment that renders this book a space in everyone's library."

> —**Perry D. Hoffman, PhD**, president and cofounder
> of National Education Alliance for Borderline
> Personality Disorder

"Blaise Aguirre and Gillian Galen have written a compassionate, sensitive, and practical book to help individuals diagnosed with borderline personality disorder (BPD) successfully navigate everyday life challenges. I'm exceptionally proud to recommend this important book to my clients as well as their family members and friends."

> —**Amanda L. Smith, LMSW**, dialectical behavior
> therapist and treatment consultant, and author of
> *The Dialectical Behavior Therapy Wellness Planner*

T0003126

"Aguirre and Galen have written a thoughtful and practical guide for people suffering with borderline personality disorder (BPD). This book will be an important resource for clients as well as professionals and family members."

>—**Michael Hollander, PhD**, director of training at McLean 3East, assistant professor of psychology in the department of psychiatry at Harvard Medical School, and author of *Helping Teens Who Cut*

"There are few books designed to help the individual suffering from borderline personality disorder (BPD) to use cognitive behavioral therapy (CBT) and dialectical behavior therapy (DBT) tools to help get them through difficult situations. A supplement to traditional coaching and therapy, this book accomplishes that with simplicity and clarity. Aguirre and Galen have written a practical guide that will serve as a road map to help clients improve their lives, and at the same time help therapists working with some of the most challenging clients."

>—**Michael Roy, LCSW**, founder and executive director of Clearview Women's Center, a treatment center specializing in borderline personality and emotional disorders

Coping
with BPD

DBT *and* **CBT SKILLS** *to*
SOOTHE *the* **SYMPTOMS**
of **BORDERLINE**
PERSONALITY DISORDER

Blaise Aguirre, MD
Gillian Galen, PsyD

New Harbinger Publications, Inc.

Publisher's Note

This publication is designed to provide accurate and authoritative information in regard to the subject matter covered. It is sold with the understanding that the publisher is not engaged in rendering psychological, financial, legal, or other professional services. If expert assistance or counseling is needed, the services of a competent professional should be sought.

This book is independently authored and published and is not endorsed or sponsored by or affiliated with any third party, including the various individuals and organizations who use the acronym DBT or the phrase Dialectical Behavior Therapy in their trademarks. Both of these terms are used in this book strictly in their generic meanings to identify a form of therapy that is utilized by many scholars and practitioners in the field of psychology. By way of example, this book is not endorsed by or affiliated in any way with Dr. Marsha M. Linehan, who is recognized as a pioneer in the field of Dialectical Behavior Therapy and who offers her professional services under the federally registered trademark DBT.

NEW HARBINGER PUBLICATIONS is a registered trademark of New Harbinger Publications, Inc.

New Harbinger Publications is an employee-owned company

Distributed in Canada by Raincoast Books

Copyright © 2015 by Blaise Aguirre and Gillian Galen
    New Harbinger Publications, Inc.
    5674 Shattuck Avenue
    Oakland, CA 94609
    www.newharbinger.com

Cover design by Amy Shoup; Acquired by Jess O'Brien; Edited by Marisa Solís

Library of Congress Cataloging-in-Publication Data

Aguirre, Blaise A.
  Coping with BPD : DBT and CBT skills to soothe the symptoms of borderline personality disorder / Blaise Aguirre, MD, and Gillian Galen, PsyD ; foreword by Alec Miller, PsyD.
      pages cm
  Includes bibliographical references.
  ISBN 978-1-62625-218-9 (paperback) -- ISBN 978-1-62625-219-6 (pdf e-book) -- ISBN 978-1-62625-220-2 (epub) 1. Borderline personality disorder--Treatment. 2. Acceptance and commitment therapy. 3. Dialectical behavior therapy. 4. Self-care, Health. I. Galen, Gillian. II. Title.
  RC569.5.B67A386 2013
  616.85'852--dc23   2015020074

Printed in the United States of America

25   24   23

15   14   13   12   11   10   9

This book is dedicated to my children, who have given me plenty of opportunities to practice skills, and to Lauren, who has learned to accept it when I tell her that this is my last book.

—Blaise

To Jed, for your endless support of all of my projects no matter the timing, and to Henry, my littlest teacher.

—Gillian

Historically, when individuals in weekly psychotherapy had problems they would have to wait for their next weekly session to talk about what had happened. For people who have BPD, having to wait a week to deal with a problem can seem like an eternity of suffering, and this suffering interferes with developing the skills necessary to effectively cope with real-life challenges in the moment. With the advent of dialectical behavioral therapy, or DBT, between-session skills coaching by phone or text gives those struggling with BPD a more real-time, or at least closer-to-real-time, option to access therapeutic coaching to more effectively cope with whatever is going on.

In this book, Aguirre and Galen have written fourteen chapters that contain clinical wisdom that is extremely generalizable. The content is presented in a unique format whereby they succinctly describe a problem (for example, a fight with a friend), then elaborate further on how the problem develops, and finally present the "practice," or practical ways of coping with the specific problem.

Most remarkably, the authors have captured and distilled the many unique and prominent problems individuals with BPD face. Thus, many chapters are devoted to managing intense negative emotions, including anger, sadness, jealousy, shame, loneliness, and boredom, to name a few.

Other chapters involve coping strategies for common challenges, such as procrastination, engaging in mood-dependent behavior, lashing out, and drug and alcohol urges. They also talk about how to tackle such problems as feeling unloved and fears of never getting better. Most BPD clients I have treated during the past twenty years describe these exact difficulties. Aguirre and Galen provide sound "coping" suggestions informed by DBT skills and strategies that will undoubtedly help individuals seeking immediate help as well as seasoned therapists looking for additional tools for their clinical armamentarium.

As with most other self-help books, it is important to recognize this is a supplement and not a replacement for traditional evidence-based psychotherapies, such as dialectical behavior therapy or mentalization-based therapy. My hope and expectation is that clients will keep this book at the ready for its immediately accessible suggestions for coping with the most common and challenging problems associated with BPD.

> —Alec L. Miller, PsyD
> Cofounder and clinical director at Cognitive & Behavioral Consultants, LLP White Plains, New York
> Professor of clinical psychiatry and behavioral sciences Montefiore Medical Center/ Albert Einstein College of Medicine Bronx, New York

patterns of thinking that lead to actions and the emotions that direct these thoughts, people can modify their patterns of thinking to improve their ability to cope. CBT fundamentally focuses on change. Although the application of a skill or solution to a problem is specific to the work we have done, the actual DBT skills are drawn from the work of Marsha Linehan (1993a, 1993b, 2014a, 2014b).

We want you to use this book as a guide. We have divided the book into fourteen chapters, each subdivided into specific situations typical in BPD. Although the fifty-three situations in this book are distinct, often the problems overlap. So even though there is overlap, we have divided them to make the solutions clearer.

Throughout the book we will ask you to pay attention to your *vulnerability factors*. These are the factors or life events that make you more vulnerable to a problematic behavior. These are things like drugs, poor sleep, lack of exercise, et cetera. Unless you pay attention to or be mindful of these factors, you are likely to continue to behave in the ways you always have—and if these ways cause suffering, you will continue to suffer.

Each specific situation is presented with the following headings:

The Problem: This is a brief overview of the situation you are in and the problem you are trying to solve.

What It Looks Like: In this section we illustrate the problem using real-world examples from actual people in therapy.

The Practice: Here we present specific skills and techniques that can be applied in each situation. Although the skills can be learned and used by anyone, we call it "the practice" because it takes time and lots of practice to achieve long-term success.

Checklist: We provide a brief list of questions to help keep you on track.

This book is small, and we planned it that way. Keep it with you and refer to it when you are stuck. It will help you while you're waiting for your therapist to call back, when he or she is not available, or when you would like to work on skills independently.

We have specifically and intentionally omitted two common problems that many people with BPD struggle with. We will not address suicidality and self-injury in this book. If you are struggling with either one of these it is imperative that you either (1) contact your therapist immediately or (2) go to your nearest emergency room for an urgent evaluation. However, because many of the problems highlighted in this book can lead to the emergence of suicidal thinking and self-injury urges, addressing these problems in the moment can mean that suicidal thinking and self-injury urges will be less likely to show up.

CHAPTER 1

Anger

turned out to be his cousin. In another situation, a woman wanted to end her relationship with her boyfriend because she had seen him looking through the swimsuit edition of a sport's magazine and was disgusted by his doing so. If you decide that the situation calls for a breakup, can you maintain your dignity and self-respect in doing so? You should also ask yourself whether the reason for breaking up is consistent with your values. Does someone looking through a magazine go against your values?

- **Validate your anger.** Whether or not you break up with the person, validating that you were angry in the moment is important. If you do end up breaking up, recognize that what happened was not *only* your fault. Most of these situations are transactional, meaning that both people in the situation have a role to play in the interaction.

- **Check your urge to blame yourself.** All too often people with BPD end up blaming themselves, which reinforces the belief that they are terrible people. So check the urge to blame yourself.

Checklist

☐ Have you taken a time out?

☐ Do you have all the facts? What was the other person's perspective?

☐ Is the reason you are breaking up in keeping with your values?

☐ Have you validated your emotions?

☐ Have you checked the urge to blame yourself?

2 · Fighting with Parents

The Problem

You and your parents are fighting. You sense that they do not trust you to make good decisions. You are angry and feel that they don't care.

What It Looks Like

Jennifer is a thirty-one-year-old who has a decent relationship with her parents. However, Jennifer feels that she can't talk to her mother about important matters, because this is typically when they start arguing. Her mother brings up Jennifer's past mistakes, which leads Jennifer to believe that her mother doesn't trust her to make her own decisions. Recently, Jennifer was offered a promotion at work. She shared the news with her mother, and they ended up arguing. "She thinks I'm a total screwup," says Jennifer. "When she told me to talk to my therapist about accepting the new job, I just wanted to explode. If she really cared about me, she would be excited for me, trust that I can make this decision, and stop reminding me of all the jobs that haven't worked out or that I have quit when I felt overwhelmed. I know that I have made mistakes in the past, but I just want to scream at her or maybe stop talking to her completely. But when I do that, I just prove her right that I can't handle myself. Sometimes I hate her, and other times I hate myself."

The Practice

Not feeling like your parents trust you, and being reminded about past failures, can be a painful experience. In these situations you may feel tremendous anger at your parents, or you may notice other emotions arise, such as feelings of regret, sadness, guilt, or shame. If you are not mindful of these emotions they can quickly get away from you, and you may find yourself lashing out at your parents and yourself. That can be a dangerous cycle, which puts you at great risk for making your situation worse and appearing—again—like you cannot be trusted to manage your emotions. Avoid this cycle by trying the following techniques:

- **Know your emotional state.** Before you can be effective with your parents, you need to take notice of what you are feeling. This is part of *mindfulness*, which is the intentional act of paying attention to the present moment without judging it. Pause to notice your rising emotions *and* the urges that accompany the emotions. If you are not aware, you are at risk of being thrown around, especially by your anger. Being mindful takes practice.

  Begin with noticing what you are feeling in your body. When you are angry, it is common to experience muscle tension, clenching of your fists, grinding of your teeth, feeling hot or flushed, or your heart beating faster. If you notice that you are angry, it is important to remind yourself that your anger is acceptable and makes sense. Remember to pay attention to any other emotions that arise as well. Anger can increase in intensity very quickly and make you move into action in ways that may not be effective.

- **Do the opposite of your urge.** The key here is to notice your urges to act and then do the opposite (Linehan 1993a,

1993b). With anger, it is most common to want to lash out. Therefore, try doing the opposite: Perhaps gently push away from the situation. Politely ask to take a break and do something else—such as going for a walk, calling a friend, or taking a cold shower—and then return to the conversation with your parents when you are feeling less angry.

Another opposite action is to practice loving compassion and do something kind for the person you feel anger toward. Exercising loving compassion takes practice and typically works best if you do so after you have excused yourself and distracted yourself for a short period of time. You may be surprised how much doing something kind for your mom or dad can change your mood. It is important to remember that you must validate your emotions before you practice an opposite action.

- **Pay attention to the content of your thinking.** Another important part of this practice is to notice your thoughts. Jennifer found herself making a very common thinking error that often occurs when one becomes upset. As Jennifer became angrier with her mother, she had the thought, "If she really cared about me she would be excited for me." Have you ever found yourself thinking this way? This is a thinking error that causes tremendous suffering, quickly increases anger, and leads to loneliness and despair.

  The error in Jennifer's thinking is that she is grasping onto one piece of data to determine if her mother cares about her. The word "if" is a helpful prompt in catching this type of error. When you notice this type of thinking, check the facts. Broaden your awareness and think about your relationship as a whole, not just this most recent interaction, before your draw an absolute conclusion.

Checklist

☐ Have you been mindful of the early signs of your anger and your action urge?

☐ Which opposite action will you do?

☐ Have you checked the facts about your relationship?

3 · Fighting with Friends

The Problem

Your group of girlfriends has started to disband from a weekly dinner get-together because some of them have found boyfriends. You are afraid that the group is going to disband and that you will be left alone without your friends. When your best friend tells you that she too has met someone, it is more than you can take and you are furious at her sudden lack of availability.

What It Looks Like

Jennel is twenty-one years old and has been with her group of friends since high school. Although many went away to college, she and five of her closest friends attended the local community college. Since senior year of high school, every Friday night they meet at one of their houses and cook dinner together. Jennel feels connected to them, and although much of the rest of her world is in turmoil, the predictable dinner nights feel like an anchor in the chaos. Elsewhere in her life she fights with her parents, has disastrous dates, and is in constant fear of losing her job because she believes that her coworkers don't like her.

When one of the six starts dating and gives up the Friday ritual, everyone is unsettled but happy for the friend. Soon others begin serious dating as well, but when Jennel's best friend says she can no longer come on Friday because she has met someone, Jennel loses it. She refuses to speak to any of them. She believes they're disloyal and selfish. When they call to check in on her, Jennel is cold at best. One

Friday night she calls her best friend and tells her that she can't stand her anymore because of all the hurt she has caused by picking a man she has known for just two months over a relationship of six years, then Jennel tells her never to call again. She then sends her dinner group an e-mail asking them to never contact her again and letting them know that she's deleting their numbers from her phone. Finally, she goes to bed and cries herself to sleep.

The Practice

If you have BPD, seeing the close friends in your life drift away and not seem to have time for you can feel so painful that it can seem as though you have lost them forever. The danger in believing that they have been intentionally hurtful is that you might do things that worsen the relationship to the point that they won't want to spend any time with you in the future. Here are some steps to dealing with fights with friends:

- **Do nothing.** You don't want to bang back when you are emotionally upset, because you will tend to be ineffective when your emotions are high; the likelihood is that you will say things out of anger. Give it some time. Avoid communicating until your anger and sadness are manageable. On the other hand, don't wait so long that you begin to catastrophize and create problems that don't exist. Once you are more settled, reach out to your friends, apologize for whatever part of the fight you were responsible for, and say that you want to talk to find a way to fix things.

- **Collect data.** Reflect on how you got to where you are by gathering evidence of your friendships. You might want to read past e-mails, text messages, or letters from your friends. You might want to look at photographs of the great times you experienced together. It is important to put the current fight in the context of the entire relationship.

- **Apologize and forgive.** It takes courage to apologize and show compassion to forgive. Both of these are marks of a dedicated friend. The forgiveness also has to be toward yourself. Beating yourself up over what has happened will only end up making you feel worse.

- **Consider where your friends are coming from.** Try to look at it from their perspective. When you speak to them, ask if they can see where you're coming from. The fight is a function of not agreeing with each other; seeing each other's perspective will allow the situation to make some sense.

- **Don't make things worse.** Don't try to make your friends jealous or angry. For instance, don't suddenly drop your group to hang out with other people with the intention of making them jealous. Not only is that hurtful to your long-time friends, it will make the new group of pals feel used.

- **Be willing to fix the problem.** Things may not return to the way they used to be, but be open to other solutions. For instance, Jennel might propose getting together once a month instead of every Friday, if that's easier for the group to commit to.

Checklist

☐ Have you given yourself some time before reacting?

☐ Have you looked at the relationship from a long-term perspective?

☐ Are you willing to apologize and forgive?

☐ Are you willing to work on alternative solutions? If so, are there some you can offer?

4 · Fighting with Coworkers

The Problem

Work can be a particularly challenging place because changing roles, differing ideas, and new personnel can lead to difficult relationships and intense emotions. When work is stressful, you might have the urge to lash out at a colleague, but this can be overwhelming and potentially job threatening.

What It Looks Like

Karl, a twenty-six-year-old software engineer with BPD, has finally found his niche at a new start-up. He feels happier than he has in a while. He makes sure to leave work at a decent time to get home, exercise, and then get to bed on time. On weekends Karl spends quality time with his girlfriend.

Lately, Karl has been hearing from his coworkers that he is not working hard enough. They tell Karl that they are staying later at the office and working on weekends, and that he doesn't seem to care enough to work as hard as they do. Although he had signed on for forty hours a week, he is already clocking sixty hours. Karl feels that he is being unfairly targeted. He notices his fury rising. Then his anger surges further—he wants to go to work and tell everyone to go to hell. He particularly wants to punch a smug programmer colleague who does not have his talent but who gets along well with their boss. This colleague seems to be the one spearheading the effort to tell Karl how little he is working.

The Practice

Research shows that 30 percent of executives and employees argue with a coworker at least once a month (Fierce Inc. 2013). When you feel angry and have the urge to lash out, try the following skills:

- **Address the conflict as soon as possible.** To prevent the issue from festering, calmly speak up and directly converse with the other person about the situation. Waiting for your coworker to apologize assumes that he knows that he has done something wrong.

- **Invite your colleague to talk about what is going on.** If you cannot do this at work, or if doing it at work will lead to escalation, then find some neutral location outside of work.

- **Be open to your colleague's point of view.** It is possible that you have only one perspective and that you are missing important information. Listen to what he has to say.

- **Define your objective.** What is the outcome that you want? Do you want to repair your relationship with your colleague? Do you simply want to vent and let him know how angry you are? Do you want to set specific limits on your coworker's behavior?

- **Get help.** You won't be able to solve all your conflicts on your own. You may need help from a supervisor, and if that does not get resolution, you may need help from the human resources department. A neutral third party will typically facilitate the finding of a solution rather than pushing a specific agenda. However, keep in mind that an HR person holds the interest of the company above your specific request.

Checklist

☐ Are you addressing the conflict without allowing it to fester?

☐ Have you invited your colleague to meet with you to try to solve the issue?

☐ Are you clear about your objective?

☐ Have you asked for help from a neutral third party?

5 · FIGHTING WITH YOUR THERAPIST

The Problem

You feel that your therapist has not been paying attention to you. You are angry at her and believe that she doesn't care about you. You feel that your sessions haven't been productive. You want to yell at her even though you know it won't make things better.

What It Looks Like

Gwen is a twenty-year-old college student who has a difficult time scheduling appointments with her therapist. In part, this has to do with Gwen's class schedule, but it also is a result of her therapist taking on additional patients. The past few therapy sessions have dealt with this reduction in access, which, for Gwen, has been difficult. In her recent session, Gwen spent most of the time crying and occasionally yelling at her therapist, including telling her that she was only doing it for the money and that she was unqualified to be a therapist. After two years of regular, weekly therapy, Gwen now feels uncared for, disconnected, and no longer a priority. After leaving the session, Gwen feels terrible. She feels that dropping out of therapy or canceling the next session is what she needs to do. She can't face more fighting, but she thinks that it is what is going to end up happening.

    One of the most difficult moments in therapy, and yet one that is inevitable, is that things will change between you and your therapist. Reasons for this stem from changes in your life, like getting a job; changing your academic schedule; moving to a new apartment; and so on. There will also be changes in your therapist's life. She may get married, have a baby, reduce her work hours, increase her workload, go on vacation, and more. Such life events may lead to a strain on the therapeutic relationship because of feelings of abandonment. In many situations, rather than processing the change in the relationship and validating the ensuing feelings, you get angry—and when this happens it can lead to fights with the therapist.

The Practice

From a DBT perspective, even though it's true that all conflicts are transactional events between two people, the only behavior that you can really manage is your own. You cannot manage your therapist's life or behavior. Ultimately, the two main components you can manage are your feelings and the actual matter you are fighting about. However, you cannot effectively manage the situation if your emotions are high.

Here are steps to avoid fighting with your therapist:

- **Notice your urge to fight.** If you are unsettled or anxious, or feel anger starting to rise before going to therapy or calling your therapist, take a moment to notice these cues. These are your urges to take actions you might regret.

- **Review your goals.** Decide whether having a fight with your therapist is consistent with your long-term goals. Also hold in mind what your goals are with regard to your relationship with your therapist.

- **Prep for your discussion.** Having a plan of action can help the session with your therapist go smoothly. Ask a trusted friend, colleague, or parent for help in figuring out exactly what to say; include role-playing with your trusted helper.

- **Be clear and concise.** Once you are back in control, when you have in mind your personal goals and have established a course of action, be clear with your therapist about what the specific situation is. For instance, saying, "I feel sad that you are taking three months of maternity leave" is far clearer and more effective than saying, "You are a terrible therapist who doesn't care about me."

Checklist

☐ Have you noticed emotions arise? Have you identified your action urge?

☐ Is having a fight with your therapist consistent with your long-term goals?

☐ Have you established what your goal is in your relationship with your therapist?

☐ Do you have a plan for how you are going to deal with the conflict?

☐ Can you role-play your action plan with a friend, including trouble-shooting what might go wrong with your plan?

6 · Wanting to Yell at People

The Problem

Several times throughout the day you interact with people you want to yell at: poor drivers, inept salespeople, noisy neighbors, lazy coworkers. You feel that people should be more organized and fair. You become angry and want to yell when you are put on phone call holds for a long time, or when you have to wait longer than a restaurant hostess predicted.

What It Looks Like

Harold, an extremely sensitive forty-four-year-old with BPD, procrastinated doing his taxes. The day before they were due, his boss badgered him repeatedly about taking initiative with a new client, and then he stayed up all night to work on them, smoking marijuana to keep calm. He fights traffic to get to the post office and then has to wait in a long line. When he hands the post office clerk the envelope, the clerk tells him that he filled out the wrong form for registered mail. The clerk asks Harold to come back to the counter when has has completed the correct form, and then he takes the next person in line. Harold feels like he's going to explode. He wants to yell at the clerk about how unfair it is that he can't be taken immediately and about how disorganized the post office is.

The Practice

Because people with BPD are more sensitive than most, plus have a reduced ability to tolerate frustration, situations in which they feel that things are unfair can rapidly escalate to them letting others know exactly how they feel—at volume. Here is how you can address the urge to yell at someone:

- **State your goals.** The first step in dealing with a situation where nothing feels more "right" than to yell at someone is to take a step back and ask yourself what your goal is. Unfortunately, it often feels that you don't have the luxury of reflection because the urge to yell seems to come up so suddenly and the impulse to do it is so irresistible. If you can, notice all the high-vulnerability factors before the situation becomes a *situation.* Is this the right time to apply for a job? Are you in the right space to ask for a raise? Are you thinking that you are ready to bite someone's head off? What can you do? Remember your goals when you answer.

- **Leave before you act.** Recognize that you are about to do something that may feel good in the moment but will end up with you looking irrational and out of control. You will likely yell things that you're going to regret, and you may have to deal with the person again.

- **Regroup before dealing with the situation again.** When you leave a frustrating situation, you still have to go back and face it. Doing so from a point of lower irritability will give you a better chance of reaching your goal. Prepare yourself by going for a walk, getting grounded, and taking a deep breath before facing the situation again.

- **Identify the actual problem.** Be clear in identifying the problem, as this will help you identify a solution. It's probably not the other person's fault. And don't blame yourself, as you are not the problem either. We all tend to blame ourselves and other people for situations we are in rather than accepting that we are in it and that we have to deal with it as effectively as we can. In Harold's situation, the problem was not the post office clerk. It was that he had left his taxes till the last moment and then did not sleep. He should solve the problem by tackling the issue of procrastinating. He shouldn't attack the person; attacking another person will not solve the problem.

- **Remember that others are watching.** Don't forget that your behavior will impact relationships and how others see you. This includes coworkers, employers, friends, strangers, and children. Is yelling how you want to represent yourself?

Checklist

☐ Leave before you yell!

☐ Regroup before tackling the situation again.

☐ Have you identified the real problem?

☐ Have you asked yourself if yelling is how you want people to remember you?

CHAPTER 2

Other Intense Emotions

7 · Sadness

The Problem

You are feeling intensely sad. Your mood is low. You don't want to do anything. You don't want to see anyone. You might not see a point to anything.

What It Looks Like

Sanjay, a forty-nine-year-old who recently ended his second marriage, describes sadness this way: "I could not stand being sad. I felt blue and alone, and I didn't want to be with anyone. I believed that the only way I could possibly survive was to cut myself off from everyone, and yet that only intensified the feeling of sadness, even if it felt like the thing to do in the moment. I simply wanted to lie in bed all day. The result of that was plummeting further into despair. Eventually, my sadness passed, but it wasn't the isolation that had helped me survive. That only increased the sadness. Reaching out to others was my way out."

Sometimes the emotion of sadness is triggered by an interaction with someone else, and sometimes it appears to come out of the blue. It is important to recognize that sadness and depression are very different things. For instance, sadness is often associated with many negative thoughts about yourself, whereas depression is attributed to negative thoughts about everything. Sadness is not a constant emotional state; however, the medical condition of depression is a serious mental illness that has enduring low mood states with disruptions in sleep, poor appetite, hopelessness, and, at times, suicidal thoughts. (Nevertheless, prolonged feeling of sadness over days and weeks can lead to a depression.) The treatment of sadness and depression are different. The medical diagnosis of depression will often require the use of medication, whereas sadness is never treated with medication.

The Practice

The natural tendency when you are feeling sad is to withdraw, retreat, slow down, isolate yourself, and maybe cry. If you do the same things over and over when you are sad, the likelihood is that you will continue to be sad. You have to change the activities you typically do when you are sad in order to feel relief from sadness.

- **Seek self-validation.** Before you can change being sad, you have to accept that you are sad. *Self-validation* is a skill that we ask you to do over and over again throughout this book. It is a practice of accepting your internal experience as real, understandable, and acceptable. You must take the time to acknowledge your feelings and determine whether they fit the situation at hand. Once you have accepted that you are sad, you then have to decide whether you want to stay sad or change the sadness. It is also important to ask yourself if your sadness is tainted with feeling sorry for yourself, because at times the thoughts themselves can perpetuate the sadness.

- **Take time to figure out what to do.** The behaviors of sadness have some value: the tendency to slow down and want to isolate yourself is the brain's way of giving you the space and time to figure out what to do about the situation you are in. Unfortunately, most people who are sad don't see it that way and therefore don't take the time to find solutions to their sadness.

- **Act opposite to the urge.** Another way to overcome sadness is to disrupt your usual response to the emotion. So if your tendency when you are sad is to withdraw and isolate your-self, do the opposite: leave your bedroom and call a friend, for instance.

- **Act compassionately.** Do a kind act for another person with the intention of not only helping that individual but also lifting your feeling of sadness. Offering to help a colleague with a project, or a roommate with her schoolwork, or a parent run errands are good examples of acts of compassion. If that seems too much to do, actively reach out by sending a kind text or e-mail to a friend or a relative, even when it feels difficult.

- **Make a list.** When your mood is low it can be hard to come up with things to talk to your friend or loved one about. So, ahead of time, compile a list of things that you might want to talk about, things that are important to you and her. This can prevent you from falling into sadness during your conversation.

Checklist

☐ Have you self-validated?

☐ Have you identified your action urge? And if so, did you act opposite to the urge?

☐ Is there someone you care about whom you can call?

☐ Have you made a list of the things you want to talk about during your conversation?

8 · Jealousy

The Problem

Jealousy is the feeling that arises when you think you are going to lose someone you really care about to someone else. It can lead to behaviors like clinging, which can accelerate the loss of the relationship and also lead to your losing your self-respect (Linehan 1993a, 1993b).

What It Looks Like

Eric is a handsome thirty-seven-year-old man with BPD who has trouble staying in relationships because of his jealousy. During one date, Eric was sitting in a restaurant with his girlfriend when she received a text from her ex-boyfriend asking her out on a date. He became extremely jealous. In that moment, Eric felt that his girlfriend was more interested in her ex than in him. He felt unattractive and wanted to hurt her, so he picked up his phone and called a girl he had recently met at work and asked if she was free for dinner later that week. He and his girlfriend broke up soon after.

A month later, Eric was dating someone else. After three weeks into their relationship, Eric's new girlfriend had gone to visit her mother, who had suffered a stroke, in the hospital. She had turned off her phone during her stay. Eric had forgotten she was at the hospital, so when she didn't pick up he became frantic, imagining that his girlfriend was with another man. He left message after message; the first was fairly benign, but by the eighth message he was accusing her of cheating on him and saying that they should break up. Later, when she left the hospital and heard all his messages, she decided that she wanted to have nothing to do with him and his high level of jealousy. When she broke up with him, he could not bear it and began to follow her. During session he admitted, "I went to her house hoping to talk to her one night, when I saw this guy there. I hid in the bushes outside her living room and watched as she made him dinner and sat talking to him. When I saw her get up and hug him, I couldn't stand it any longer. I went up and rang the doorbell. She was surprised and introduced me to her brother. I was so ashamed that I made an excuse and left. What is happening to me? Even when I knew it was her brother, I was still jealous. Why can't I let this go?"

Eric's jealousy comes in two different forms. The first type is a reaction to things that have actually happened, which is considered *justified* jealousy. For instance, when his girlfriend received a text message invitation for a date with her ex, one could say Eric's jealousy was justified. The second type of jealousy is a reaction based on a suspicion. When there is no evidence of wrongdoing, this is *unjustified* jealousy. When Eric felt that his girlfriend was more interested in her ex than him, or when Eric made threats and accusations over voicemail when his new girlfriend didn't answer his calls, his behavior could be considered unjustified jealousy. He had no evidence that either woman had feelings for anyone else or was cheating on him.

The emotion of jealousy has characteristic thoughts and physical symptoms:

Thoughts

- *I am not as attractive as the other person.*

- *I am not as smart as the other person.*

- *I am not as important as the other person.*

- *She is cheating on me.*

- *I feel rejected.*

- *I need to get revenge.*

Physical Sensations

- Lump in your throat

- Dry mouth

- Fast heartbeat

- Suspiciousness and paranoia

As you can see from the list of thoughts, there is the fundamental feeling that you are not good enough.

The Practice

When jealousy is a justified reaction to something that has actually threatened the relationship, you should consider what is in *your* best interest. You have to decide whether it is important for you to:

- Protect the relationship you have

- Fight for your relationship, even if you fear it won't work

- Leave the relationship

If you decide that it is essential that you stay in the relationship, you will need to:

- Talk to the person you care about.

- Explain what your experience is, including your thoughts and feelings.

- Determine what can be done about the threat.

It is also possible that the relationship is not worth saving and that, in order to preserve your self-respect, you should walk away from it. Not every relationship is worth holding on to, and you have to decide whether it is truly worth it.

When jealousy is based solely on suspicion or is unjustified, it is time to practice the DBT skill of the opposite action to jealousy. You can do this by:

- Purposely sharing the person you love with others

- Avoiding stalking, snooping, and reading private texts and e-mails

- Letting go of the need to control the person you love

An important aspect to opposite action is to consider how you would have acted had you not felt jealous. Let's look at Eric's situation. In response to jealousy, instead of trying to confront his girlfriend and her brother, Eric could have done the opposite, perhaps inviting them both to dinner the next evening. Think about what opposite action could have applied in your situation.

Checklist

☐ Have you established whether your jealousy is justified or unjustified?

☐ Is this relationship truly worth saving?

☐ Have you talked to your loved one and shared your feelings?

☐ How would you be acting if you were not jealous?

9 · GUILT

The Problem

You are feeling intensely guilty. Your mood is low and you feel like an awful person who always hurts people and messes up. You hate yourself. Nothing seems to matter. The guilt is overwhelming, and you don't know what to do.

What It Looks Like

Kendra is a twenty-nine-year-old who is anxious about an upcoming interview. At home, she waits for her best friend, who has agreed to leave work a few hours early to help her prepare. However, Kendra's friend is stuck in traffic and therefore running late. As time passes, Kendra becomes more anxious about her interview and angry that her friend is late. When Kendra's friend arrives, she apologizes and then explains that there was an accident that closed the highway. Before her friend can sit down, Kendra screams, "If you cared about me you would have been here on time! What kind of friend are you? Don't you know that this is important to me? It doesn't even matter anymore—I probably won't get the job anyway. Clearly you don't think I can do it or else you would have made this a priority. Just leave!"

Kendra's devaluing behavior drives her friend to leave, and Kendra is left alone in her apartment. Her anger quickly fades and she is hit hard by an intense wave of guilt. She realizes that her friend was making a sacrifice by leaving work early and that her friend wanted to help her. Kendra's guilt deepens when she remembers all the relationships she has destroyed by engaging in this behavior.

The Practice

Guilt is a powerful emotion that many people find hard to manage. Recognizing guilt is often quite painful and leads to feelings of worthlessness, hopelessness, and, for some, a sense of toxicity. Extreme feelings of guilt can lead people to feel like life is not worth living. The natural tendency when you are feeling guilty is to retreat, withdraw, or isolate yourself, cry, get angry, and maybe punish yourself for your behavior. If you engage in those types of behaviors you will only make your guilt more intense and feel more isolated and alone. To lessen your guilt, you can work to make repairs and take care of your relationships in a way that shows a recommitment to your own values and morals. Here's how you do it:

- **Identify your values.** Guilt typically arises when you have done something that violates your values or moral code. (Although you might feel guilt *without* having violated your values, those emotions are dealt with differently; see "Let go of mistakes," below.) *Values* are your principles of behavior and things that are of importance to you. Values help you figure out how to act and what to prioritize.

  People have values around family, work, social behavior, and so on. For example, you might value honesty, being on time, exercising, or treating others the way you want to be treated. If you have trouble identifying your values by asking yourself what is important to you, there are many lists of personal values online that you may find helpful. Knowing your moral code is an important first step to changing your guilt.

- **Determine whether your guilt is justified or unjustified.**
  The next step is to determine whether the guilt you are
  feeling is justified or unjustified (Linehan 2014a, 2014b). To
  do this, ask yourself whether your behavior violates your own
  moral code or values, or whether your social group would
  reject you if they found out about your behavior. If the answer
  to either question is yes, then your guilt is likely justified. If
  neither of these conditions is true, then your guilt is unjustified. This is a very important distinction.

  For instance, Kendra's guilt is justified, since her actions
  went against her values of not devaluing friends or destroying relationships. (On the other hand, if Kendra felt guilty
  because she forgot to turn the lights off when she left home,
  she did *not* defy her values—she simply made a mistake!
  Unjustified guilt can be common in some people with BPD,
  and if this is your situation, the skills you need to use to
  change guilty feelings are different; see "Let go of mistakes,"
  later in this list.)

  With justified guilt, you must self-validate and make a
  commitment to yourself to keep working on changing your
  automatic behaviors. You may want to give up, but that will
  only make you feel worse. Again, ask yourself if a feeling of
  self-pity is making your guilt or anger at yourself more intense.
  It is easy to fall into that trap when you are feeling guilt.

- **Try an opposite action.** Managing guilt is another situation
  in which doing the opposite of your typical reaction can help
  relieve your suffering. If your guilt is justified, the opposite
  action would be to apologize and find a way to repair your
  transgression. This is a not an easy task, but it will have a
  powerful and positive impact on your mood.

- **Strategize for the future.** Make a commitment to not engage
  in the behavior again—perhaps work on a plan for how you
  will cope in a similar situation in the near future, or ask your
  therapist for help.

- **Take responsibility for your actions.** Accept the consequences of your behavior, and then use mindfulness techniques to not dwell on the events or overapologize; instead work on letting it go. It can be very easy to get stuck ruminating on behaviors you feel guilty about, but again this will only make your situation worse.

- **Let go of mistakes.** Unjustified emotions are not helpful to us, as they do not give us accurate information. If your guilt does not fit the situation—meaning that it's unjustified—it helps to expose yourself to the scenario over and over again. Using the example above, Kendra would commit to keeping the lights on when leaving home, and then practice tolerating it. This may sound strange, but with repeated practice it will help Kendra's brain begin to differentiate when guilt is warranted from when it is not. Try this practice with your own unjustified guilty feelings.

Checklist

☐ Did you engage in behaviors that violated your personal values or morals?

☐ Is your guilt justified or unjustified?

☐ Have you tried to act opposite? Did you apologize?

☐ Have you made a plan for similar future scenarios?

☐ Have you accepted the consequences of your behavior?

☐ Can you let go of any mistakes and find some self-compassion?

10 · SHAME

The Problem

You are feeling tremendous shame. It is different from feeling embarrassed or guilty, which are feelings that arise in the context of a specific behavior. Shame is an emotion that relates directly to our sense of self. It is the feeling that you are terrible or worthy of contempt, a feeling of being completely unacceptable as a human being.

What It Looks Like

Samantha is nineteen years old and struggles with feelings of shame. She feels shame for two reasons. One is that when she was six years old she was abused by her older cousin and feels that she is to blame for what happened. She tends to withdraw from any family functions that include this cousin, and she has suffered from nightmares for years. Samantha's second and more recent source of shame stems from her stealing money from a neighbor in order to buy marijuana for herself and her boyfriend. Samantha's boyfriend introduced her to marijuana a few months ago, and she found that it helped with her anxiety. But she doesn't have the money to support her habit. Samantha feels like a terrible person for stealing, but she really likes to get high with her boyfriend. She desperately wants to keep her abuse and stealing a secret; she works hard to avoid thinking about her situation and feelings.

The Practice

For many people, shame can be one of the most difficult emotions to tolerate. It often includes avoidant behaviors and secrets, both of which enhance the very feelings of shame you want relief from. The way to deal with shame is to use the skill of opposite action to reduce shame, and the first step to doing that is to determine whether the shame you are feeling is justified or unjustified. Does your behavior violate your values? Would your friends reject you if they found out about your behavior? If yes, then your shame is justified. If neither of these conditions is true, then your shame is unjustified. This is a very important distinction.

Often people with BPD suffer from a lot of unjustified shame. Samantha struggles with both. Her feelings of shame about her abuse are unjustified, as she did not cause the abuse, even if she feels that she did. (Samantha's experience is a common one for victims of abuse.) However, Samantha's feelings of shame about stealing are justified, since stealing violates her values. Justified and unjustified shame must be managed differently.

Justified Shame

When the shame is justified, use these skills:

- **Use opposite action.** Notice what you would typically do, and, if it's ineffective, do the opposite behavior.

- **Repair the transgression.** Find out how you can begin to make up for what you have done.

- **Apologize.** Do so openly and directly for whatever behavior is causing the shame.

- **Make a promise.** Commit to not doing the behavior again in the future.

- **Accept the consequences.** Take responsibility for your behavior as gracefully as possible.

- **Let it go.** Practicing mindfulness is one way to do this.

Unjustified Shame

When the shame is not justified, use these skills:

- **Repeat your behavior.** Frequently repeat the behavior that has caused the shame. Practice experiencing that feeling over and over again until the intensity reduces. This may feel counterintuitive or scary—or both. This is a very difficult skill and one that can have a powerful result when you practice it. Samantha would work with her therapist on ways to expose herself to these feelings; she may share memories or secrets that she kept about her cousin. She and her therapist would make a rank-order list of challenging situations and deal with the most difficult ones last. This is not the kind of work she would do on her own.

- **Face the trigger.** Your task is to approach, not avoid, the thing that makes you feel ashamed (Linehan 2014a, 2014b).

Checklist

☐ Did you engage in a behavior that crossed your personal values or morals?

☐ Is your shame justified or unjustified?

☐ Have you used opposite action?

☐ If your shame is justified, have you made amends and worked on letting it go?

☐ If your shame is unjustified, are you repeating the behavior?

11 · FEAR

The Problem

Fear can get in the way of setting a limit you need to set because of the worry that you will lose someone you care about. Not acting on what you need to do because of fear means that others won't know what your limits are, that they will continue to do things that bother you, and that you won't learn to overcome situations in which you are afraid.

What It Looks Like

Kathryn, a twenty-two-year-old sophomore in college, was recently hired for the evening shift as a lobby clerk at a boutique hotel. She felt happy when her parents and best friend told her how proud they were of her. Her roommate, however, was annoyed by the fact that she could no longer party with Kathryn at night. She started to send text messages to Kathryn that called her a loser and said that she would never get a boyfriend if she didn't party. Kathryn was very hurt by the texts but was terrified of setting a limit for fear of being judged by her roommate.

The Practice

There are six steps to overcoming fear:

1. **Recognize the emotion as fear.** This is the first step. It is typical and useful to experience fear in situations where a

real danger exists, because fear is an adaptive human response. Fear will usually trigger the so-called *fight-or-flight response* and prepare the mind and body to respond quickly and decisively. Physical symptoms, thoughts, and urges of fear include:

- Increasing anxiety or panic
- An intense desire to avoid or leave the situation
- Feeling "unreal" or disconnected from yourself
- Fear that you are going crazy or that you are losing your mind
- Feeling like you're going to pass out
- Thoughts that others will judge you

2. **Validate the fear.** Once you have recognized the fear, you have to determine whether it makes sense that you would have it. You are not choosing to be afraid. The fear just is. If the fear is of something that could potentially hurt you—say, you're in a room with a rattlesnake—that would be a justified fear. For Kathryn, fear of setting a limit with her roommate is an unjustified fear, since neither the limit nor her roommate is going to put her in physical danger. It makes sense that Kathryn would fear losing her friend; however, not setting the limit is not consistent with her own values.

3. **Act opposite to the fear urge.** Fear tells you that you are incapable of dealing with the situation. Standing up for yourself means challenging this way of thinking and proving the fear wrong. When you fear that you can't do something and want to run away, act opposite to the urge of backing down: challenge the fear!

4. **Don't ruminate.** If you have BPD, you may often become a prisoner of your own habitual thoughts and dwell on them.

Sometimes this type of rumination can lead to catastrophizing the situation whereby you imagine a situation much worse than the one you are facing. You are kept prisoner by playing this situation over and over again in your head. Catching the rumination and noting that it is simply a creation of your mind gives you a good chance of facing the situation more effectively than if you are paralyzed by the fear.

5. **Keep your eye on your goal.** Kathryn's goal is to keep her job and stay away from situations that are going to compromise her newfound self-respect. By knowing that this is important and consistent with her goal of healthy living, she can confidently set the limit. When you are facing a fear, remind yourself of what your goals are and of their importance to you. Don't apologize for having set your goals; they are the very things you need to move forward.

6. **Trust your instinct and act quickly.** Sometimes the fear you face is real. For instance, if you find yourself in a potentially dangerous situation, like seeing a physically abusive ex-boyfriend who's angry that you left him, and your instinct tells you to leave the situation, then leave. Sometimes your fear is unjustified, meaning that there is no factual threat. Instead, you're creating a threat in your mind—perhaps with a worry thought like *My friends hate me.* If the fear is all in your thinking, don't avoid the situation and run away. Notice the fear and deal with it as soon as is feasible. Leaving it until a much later time or avoiding it altogether will keep you stuck in suffering. If the outcome is what Kathryn fears—that her friend ends up thinking of her as a loser—then dealing with the fear immediately means that she will find out immediately. Waiting for weeks before she deals with it means that she will suffer for weeks before finding out—and then still have the outcome she feared.

Checklist

☐ Have you established that you are experiencing fear?

☐ Have you validated that your fear makes sense given the situation?

☐ Can you recognize your urge to avoid your fear and instead act opposite to it?

☐ Are you ruminating over all the possible negative outcomes?

☐ Are you keeping in mind the goals you have set for yourself and how they move your life forward?

☐ Are you listening to your own wisdom or are you procrastinating in doing what you need to do?

12 · DISGUST

The Problem

Disgust is the response you have to things you find repulsive. Some of the things that trigger disgust are inborn, like the smell of rotting food or the bitter taste of some plants; experiencing these things causes repulsion that's natural, not learned. However, there is another type of disgust that is learned—it's the disgust elicited by the behavior of others.

What It Looks Like

Scarlet is a twenty-four-year-old who is desperate to date. She's had many past relationships, but she finds sex to be repulsive. She joined an online dating site and specifically wrote that she likes kissing but does not want anyone interested in sex. Specifically, she does not like nudity or body fluids. She finally met a man who said he was a virgin and that he too was not interested in sex. After their first date they went back to her apartment, where he quickly undressed and suggested that they have sex. She was disgusted by his behavior and immediately kicked him out of her apartment.

The Practice

Here is how you overcome feelings of disgust:

- **Recognize the emotion as disgust.** Typically the disgust reaction is that your eyebrows pull down, your nose wrinkles, your upper lip is pulled up, your bottom lip is loose, and you stick out your tongue. These facial movements are the ones that precede actual retching. There can also be nausea or a sense of uneasiness in your stomach.

- **Validate the disgust.** Once you have recognized your reaction as disgust, validate that it makes sense that you would have it. If you were looking at rotten food, it would make sense that you would be repulsed by it; that's the body's way of saying, "Don't eat that or you'll get sick." When your disgust is elicited by someone else's behavior, an important practice is to decide whether it crosses your moral values.

   Now, just because it may go against your moral values does not mean that the behavior is immoral. You shouldn't trust disgust to give you reliable information about the morality of an action; however, you can validate that the behavior is something that disgusts you. Behaviors vary from one culture to the next, and what a person from another culture does may disgust you. Notice the fact that something that disgusts you may be acceptable elsewhere, and yet it is still valid that the behavior disgusts you.

- **Act opposite to the disgust urge.** In Scarlet's case, she decided that she had to overcome her disgust reaction to sex, particularly after she met a man who respected her value system and complied with her request to not engage in sex. She noticed becoming more attracted to him and eventually more aroused by him. She decided that she didn't want to connect sex with disgust. Her feelings of disgust served no purpose and prevented her from getting close to someone she felt love for.

   The only way to change the feeling of disgust is to repeatedly expose yourself to the repulsion until you reach the point at which you can tolerate it without being disgusted by it. Eventually Scarlet managed this by imagining being married to a man she met and started to date, and one day having a family with him. She also agreed to exposure to sex. She did not want to have sex immediately with her boyfriend for fear that the disgust would make her feel repulsed by him. Instead she watched very erotic movies and eventually some porn until she no longer found sexual activity repulsive.

Another example of how this works is when some parents of newborns are initially repulsed by their child's dirty diapers; however, over time they become less and less so, even though they may be disgusted by the dirty diapers of other people's children.

Checklist

☐ Have you established that you are experiencing disgust?

☐ Have you validated that your disgust makes sense given your past experiences and beliefs?

☐ Can you recognize your urge to turn away from the situation and act opposite to the disgust urge?

☐ Are you equating your disgust with moral disagreement?

☐ Are you willing to expose yourself to the situation over and over again?

CHAPTER 3

Loneliness

13 · FEARING ABANDONMENT

The Problem

You fear that people close to you are going to leave you. You believe that you are too much of a burden for them. It makes sense to you that they would want to leave you.

What It Looks Like

John is a thirty-four-year old man who is afraid that his wife is going to leave him. He gets angry at her then begs for her forgiveness; this pattern has been going on for years. For some time she has wanted a baby, but in recent months she has said that she is not certain anymore. John is worried that this is the end of the relationship.

In such situations we see two patterns of behavior. One is that John may bend over backward and do everything he can to keep her from leaving. The problem with this approach is that he might compromise his values or needs and not articulate his legitimate concerns. The second pattern is that he might hold on to her far too tightly. He might start to monitor her calls, read her text messages, check her e-mails, and follow her car. He might become jealous of her other friendships and prevent her from seeing others. He could become extremely angry and say hurtful and devaluing things when he feels that she is not prioritizing him.

This is precisely the behavior that burns out many partners and prompts them to want to leave. This is because many partners feel threatened by such behavior. They feel angry at the lack of trust in the relationship. Unfortunately, at times a person who fears abandonment will go to the extreme of trying to control his partner's behavior, thoughts, and emotions, sometimes through intimidation, threats of self-harm, or even violence. This would then lead to the very action that John fears: his wife leaving him. It can become a self-fulfilling prophecy in that in future relationships the pattern of fearing abandonment leads to overcontrolling behavior, and then the loved one leaves because she cannot tolerate the degree of jealousy and rageful behavior.

The Practice

Here is how you overcome the fear of abandonment:

- **Recognize you have this fear.** Are you clinging on too tight, feeling jealous, afraid the other person is cheating on you, becoming rageful when she doesn't seem to be prioritizing you, or fearing that she is going to leave?

- **Identify your abandonment behaviors.** What are your specific behaviors? What are your specific emotions? What are your specific thoughts? Write all of these down to help you know your pattern.

- **Identify triggers and vulnerability factors.** What behaviors in the other person are triggering your fear? Is the fear worse at night when you are tired? Are you using substances that are clouding your thinking? Have you had other relationships that have ended in a similar way? Be clear about the specific facts, and don't confuse your fears for facts.

- **Communicate directly with your loved one.** Let the other person know that you recognize the fear. Let her know that you are paying attention to your behavior, and be explicit as to what your needs, wants, and goals are. Be clear that you want to change your behavior. Own it as your problem. Ask your loved one for reasonable help with diminishing your fear triggers. For instance, you might say, "If you know you are going to be late, please call. If you have an unexpected work commitment, please acknowledge how difficult your absence is for me and send me a text." It is not your loved one's responsibility to solve your fear of abandonment; however, if she values your relationship and can validate your fear, she should be able to respond in a supportive way.

- **Act opposite to your urge.** All the recognition without behavioral change will be of little use, so this is the most important step. When you notice the fear of abandonment, rather than acting on the feeling, give your loved one the benefit of the doubt: act lovingly toward her, or go for a walk instead of getting on the phone and blasting her. Do the opposite of whatever relationship-destroying behavior you would typically do.

Checklist

☐ Have you identified and articulated the fear?

☐ Have you communicated clearly with your loved one?

☐ Have you recognized what your behavior urge is?

☐ Act opposite to this behavioral urge.

14 · FEELING LONELY

The Problem

Sometimes you just feel lonely. Everyone you normally spend time with and talk to is either not around or not available. This loneliness feels unbearable, and all you want is to feel less lonely.

What It Looks Like

Catherine is a successful thirty-two-year-old creative director with lots of friends and a supportive husband. When she became pregnant, she carefully planned a one-year leave of absence to take care of her first baby, something she has always wanted to do and believes is important to her child's development. But after three months of being a stay-at-home mom, Catherine is feeling particularly lonely. Her coworkers get to collaborate on exciting design projects without her, her friends regularly go out drinking and dancing, and her husband has picked up an extra shift at work, so she only sees him a few hours every day. Despite being with her baby around the clock, she feels a deep sense of loneliness that she can barely tolerate.

The Practice

Here is how you address the feeling of being lonely:

- **Call someone you care about.** There are people in our lives who care about us, and whom we care about, but we forget to reach out and let them know. Call them and find out what they are doing—and catch them up on how you are doing.

- **Pick three friends and knit them a scarf.** You can even make the act of knitting a mindfulness practice. In doing something kind for these friends, you will see how much they appreciate your effort when you give it to them. If knitting is outside your skill set, make them a personalized card and tell them how much you care about them.

- **Get off social media sites.** We hear over and over again from people with BPD who visit sites like Facebook and Instagram and get enraged when they see their friends having fun. Very rarely do people post the "bad stuff" or a poor picture of themselves! Ask yourself if being on social media is making you happier. If so, fine. However, you also have to pay attention to when it makes you feel more lonely and isolated—and then take a break from it when these feelings arise.

- **Volunteer.** Volunteering is not only a way to meet like-minded people, it's also a way to contribute to the happiness of others.

- **Cry.** People with BPD have a hard time self-validating. Crying without judging your crying is a great way to self-validate. Choose a period of time to cry and set a timer, because you don't want to spend the whole day crying!

- **Exercise.** Going to the gym, going to the yoga studio, or joining a soccer or running club not only makes you feel better and gets you healthy, it also gives you the opportunity to meet people, which is an effective way to broaden your social network and meet people who have similar interests. If these seem like big commitments, try building a fifteen-minute walk into your daily routine.

- **Befriend a pet.** Consider getting a pet, or spend more time with the one you already have. If you don't own a pet, consider taking care of someone else's pet for a week or so. Or go to a local pet store or an animal protection organization or shelter to play with their animals. See if spending time with animals makes you feel less lonely.

- **Join a club.** If you have a particular interest in dance, singing, poetry, photography, reading, writing, or another activity, look to see if there are clubs that meet in your local area. Using the example above, Catherine could join a club for stay-at-home moms or a parent network.

Checklist

☐ Have you identified and articulated the fear around your loneliness?

☐ Have you communicated clearly with your loved ones or reached out to a friend?

☐ Does turning off your social network feeds make you feel less lonely?

☐ Have you joined a club, started volunteering, or began exercising?

15 · FEELING BORED

The Problem

Feeling bored is an unpleasant state of being. It can make time drag on, and then when this happens, your mind can start to wander. For people with BPD, a wandering mind can tend to go to some pretty self-destructive and self-judging places.

What It Looks Like

Marco is a a bright seventeen-year-old high-school junior who hates weekends. This is because he loves to study and be at school, and he dislikes having nothing to do on the weekend. He notices dread on Thursday night, and by Friday he is quite irritable. If he had the option, Marco says that he "would sleep the entire weekend away" because he can't seem to find his way out of boredom.

It's not that there is a lack of things to do. In fact, when we ask him what he could do, Marco rattles off ten activities. His list even includes things he wants to do, like watching movies, reading books, and listening to music. Yet Marco struggles with boredom.

The Practice

Here are ways you can combat feelings of boredom:

- **Define the problem.** What is it that you are experiencing? Is it a lack of interest in everything? Or is it that you don't have the motivation to do the things that you normally want to do? Is it that there are truly no activities at all available to you? Or that you can't think of anything to do? If the latter is the case, perhaps getting advice from a friend could help.

- **Rule out other emotions.** If you're feeling a state of avoidance, or loneliness, or self-judgment, the solution is not as simple as just doing something, because you may not be experiencing boredom but instead another mind state. Be clear about what you mean by boredom. For instance, you might say, "I am feeling uncared for," or "I worry that no one wants to do anything with me," or "I hate myself and can't imagine that anyone likes me either."

- **Make a list of interesting activities.** Your list might include cooking, joining a book club, playing cards, being with friends, drawing, studying, playing a sport, or lying by the pool. Make sure that your list has a range of activities; for instance, you can't lie by the pool in the middle of winter, so be certain there are a few indoor or cold-weather options on it as well.

- **Expand your repertoire.** If you only have one or two things that seem to interest you, then take up some other activity. Learn to play the guitar, try martial arts, experiment with knitting, or learn a new language. The more activities you have in your anti-boredom kit, the more likely you are to find a solution to feeling bored.

- **Solve the actual problem.** Once you have determined that it is actual boredom that you're feeling, then engage fully in one or more of the activities or pursuits on your list. But if you have been labeling every experience that you don't like as "boredom," then look to other sections in this book for exercises to address the true problem you may be having, such as self-judgment or avoidance.

Checklist

☐ Have you defined what you mean by boredom?

☐ If it is not actual boredom that you're feeling, have you addressed the true problem?

☐ Have you created a list of interests?

☐ Do you have ideas of how you might expand your repertoire?

16 · MISSING SOMEONE IMPORTANT TO YOU

The Problem

You deeply miss your best friends and family, now that they've moved away for college, work, or other major commitments. It feels like you have no control and that no one can replace them. You feel alone and long for them desperately, almost painfully.

What It Looks Like

Carlos is nineteen, and after graduating from high school all of his best friends moved away. He had chosen to go to school locally so that he could continue to see his therapist and be closer to his parents, who are a source of great support to him. Nevertheless, he feels so alone that it's painful to even think of his friends. It is worse when he sees their pictures on Facebook, as they all seem to be having great fun; at times Carlos feels that they have completely forgotten him.

Practice

Whether for a best friend, an ex-love, or a relative who is no longer immediately in your life, deep, longing feelings are hard to bear. The first step to managing your feelings is to determine whether this person you miss so much is someone you plan on keeping in your life. For instance, you may decide that your father, who has remarried and moved to another state, is definitely a fixture in your life; however, a high school ex-boyfriend, who is now dating someone else at college, might be someone you decide to let go. Think carefully about your relationship with the person you are missing, and decide whether you see him in your future.

If you miss someone who will remain in your life, take the following actions:

- **Stay in touch.** If your loved one has moved away, set up different ways to stay in regular contact. You could arrange a weekly call or video-chat session. You might plan your vacations so that they include visits to see your loved one.

- **Listen to music that reminds you of the other person.** Create a playlist of your loved one's favorite music, or of music that you listened to together. It will likely make you sad, which is a valid response, yet doing this will allow you to connect to sadness. If you break down and cry, this is self-validating and a far better experience than numbing out or becoming angry. Because it is self-validating, after you cry or experience sadness you will feel more connected and experience more peace and calm.

- **Write your loved one a letter.** Rather than sending a text or interacting via social media, sit down with pen and paper and write the person a letter. Share your experience, thank him for the joy he brings to your life, list the things you learned from him, and convey your appreciation for him being in your life. You might want to share a specific memory that captures the bond between you.

- **Stay active.** Moping around thinking about how much you miss your loved one won't bring him back, and in all likelihood he would not want you to do that. Stay busy: watch comedies on TV, garden, or cook. This could also be a great opportunity for you to pick up a new hobby such as yoga, tennis, playing the piano, or knitting.

- **Meet new people.** You can never replace your family or old friends, but you can certainly make new connections. Extend an invitation to someone new at your work or school, or make an effort to spend time with a group that seems interesting. It may be difficult, at first, to feel accepted, but asking people about themselves is a great way to get them interested in you. Making new friends will lessen the impact of missing the people who have moved away.

If you miss someone who will not remain in your life, the following can help you move forward:

- **Validate your emotions.** If you miss a romantic partner after a breakup, especially if the relationship was intense, moving on will be one of the hardest things to do. Let yourself feel the emotions that you feel. If you need to cry, be angry, or be confused, simply allow yourself the time to experience all of these. Saying that you shouldn't feel any of these feelings will make it take longer to let go of the person.

- **Get rid of physical reminders.** If the person has truly moved on from your life—and you from his—and yet you are still in pain, get rid of everything that makes you think of him: old photos, clothes, letters, e-mails, and texts. If the memento is valuable, like jewelry, you may want to sell it or donate it to a favorite charity. Alternatively, you can give the item to a trusted other to hold on to until you are in a place to deal with everything.

- **Don't make contact.** Maintaining contact with a person you decided will not remain in your life will make it more difficult to overcome the pain of your sorrow. Don't call, text, e-mail, or connect through social media. If you have common friends, ask that they not bring up the other person. If seeing him is unavoidable, such as at work or school, then be cordial without expressing much emotion and move on to your next obligation.

- **Change your routine.** Stop doing many of the things you did together, and don't frequent the places you went together, like restaurants or parks, as long as these activities and locations continue to bring sorrow. This also allows you to take control of doing things that you may have wanted to do in the past but might not have been able to do because of this person.

Checklist

☐ Have you determined whether this person will remain in your life or not?

☐ If so, have you determined ways to stay connected even though he is far away?

☐ If he won't continue to be in your life, are you doing things to let him go?

17 · MISSING YOUR THERAPIST

The Problem

Your therapist has just gone on maternity leave and you are noticing fear and panic. You worry that she might not come back. You miss her and don't particularly like the therapist who is covering for her. You spend a lot of time talking to the covering therapist about how much you miss your regular therapist.

What It Looks Like

Eunice is a thirty-five-year-old accountant who finally decided to get herself into therapy after a string of failed romantic relationships. After eight months of helpful therapy sessions that resulted in her first relationship that lasted for more than two months, her therapist announced that she was pregnant. Five months later, the therapist went on maternity leave, and Eunice agreed to work with her therapist's office mate for the duration of the leave.

Eunice really missed her therapist. She started to notice that every day seemed like an eternity. Every time she went to therapy, the office reminded her of her old therapist, and she began to resent the covering therapist for not being her regular therapist. What bothered Eunice even more were thoughts that her therapist would never return; she even had feelings of jealousy toward the baby.

Practice

If you are missing your therapist, you can try the following:

- **Notice all-or-nothing thinking and rumination.** In the depths of despair, it is easy to imagine that your therapist will never come back. Maternity leave is often the most difficult for patients because it is the longest. Vacations are also difficult, as are unexpected absences due to illness or other events in the therapist's private life.

  If possible, get a clear sense of just how long your therapist is going to be away. For instance, maternity leave is typically three months. Even though three months can feel like an eternity, and you might believe she is never coming back, you will prolong your own suffering by spending a lot of time ruminating on her absence. Once you have noticed your rumination and all-or-nothing thinking, do other activities to help distract you. Spend time with friends and build on those and other relationships.

- **Listen to her voicemail greeting.** It may seem trivial, but hearing your therapist's away message can help trigger fond memories and keep them in your mind.

- **Keep a memento.** Therapists will sometimes give their patients a permanent or temporary object or gift to remind their patients of them. For instance, your therapist may give you her favorite pen, the one she uses when she takes notes in sessions. Or she might write you a note that you can read whenever the feeling of missing her is particularly strong, or she could record an encouraging message on your phone. Such a memento would be something to prearrange if the absence is planned. If the absence is due to a sudden illness, reading a book that your therapist recommended would be another way to have a shared object.

- **Honor the work that you have done together.** Little makes a therapist happier than to return to the work that you have done together and find out that you have continued to make gains. Having the covering therapist rave about your work during your therapist's absence is exactly the kind of reward that will keep your regular therapist wanting to continue to work with you. A client going back to old behaviors is disheartening for a therapist and will make a therapist question the value of the progress you have made.

- **Continue to make progress with your covering therapist.** You might go on a mini-strike and decide that you are not going to do any "real" work while your therapist is away. You might choose not to take therapy as seriously in working with the covering therapist. This position will simply keep you miserable. Ultimately, you are doing the work for yourself and not for your therapist. Staying stuck or freezing your progress in the place that you left off with your therapist will not get you closer to your long-term therapeutic goals. Your covering therapist may not know you as well as your regular therapist does, but he might offer alternative perspectives and new ideas that could be useful in your recovery. Be open to different suggestions.

Checklist

☐ Have you noticed rumination?

☐ Are you honoring the work you and your regular therapist have done together?

☐ Do you have a memento or voice message that is useful?

☐ Are you continuing to work proactively in therapy?

CHAPTER 4

Observing Personal Limits

18 · Saying No

The Problem

It can be very difficult for you to say no to others' requests. You might be afraid that you are being rude, or that you have the reputation of always saying yes to uphold, or that you simply don't want to fight with the other person. Sometimes people with BPD don't say no because they worry that the other person will think poorly of them or even abandon them; in turn, the person with BPD does things that cross his values.

What It Looks Like

Seth is a twenty-two-year-old gay man with BPD. He only recently came out to his friends and family and has since been introduced to other single gay men, even though he hadn't asked to be set up. He wanted to take the whole dating scene slowly, but all his friends were excited, and Seth didn't want to say no and disappoint them. One of the people he was introduced to was a much older man who seemed nice at their introduction but soon started calling Seth and insisting on a date. Seth went reluctantly to dinner and soon after ended up at the older man's house. The man insisted on sex, a request that made Seth very uncomfortable. He wanted to say no but didn't know how. It was against his values to be intimate with someone he had just met and to be forced into something that he did not want to do. But not knowing how to say no, he went along. The whole experience was emotionally and physically miserable.

The Practice

The FAST skill of DBT (Linehan 1993a, 1993b) is a powerful way to say no. FAST is an acronym that stands for: be **F**air, no **A**pologies, **S**tick to your values, and be **T**ruthful. Expanding on the FAST skill, we have come up with be **CLEAR** when you say no:

Communicate directly. Make clear statements like "No, I cannot do what you are asking," or "No, that is not something I am going to do."

Lying will lead to guilt. Don't lie.

Excuses and apologies are not necessary. Don't apologize for saying no.

Act now. It is better to say no now and deal with the situation than to be resentful later.

Respect yourself. Your self-worth does not depend on what you do for others.

Other ideas include:

- **Practice saying no.** Go over the scenario with a friend and rehearse saying no.

- **Say what you mean.** Don't say things like "I'll think about it" if you mean no. This delays what you have to do and will make you even more stressed until you say no.

Checklist

☐   Have you been clear to the other person?

☐   Are you making excuses or apologizing?

☐   Are you sticking to your values?

☐   Are you acting now?

19 · Asking for What You Need

The Problem

Communication is an essential skill, particularly when you want something out of a situation. Sometimes you may not get what you want because what you want is not possible for the other person to give. Other times you might not get what you want because very strong emotions get in the way, and either you are ineffective in how you are asking, or the strong emotions distract from a reasonable request. It is important to remember that even the most skillful people don't always get what they want, and that accepting the answer no in a manner that doesn't make the situation worse is, in and of itself, a skillful way to manage situations.

What It Looks Like

Dustin is a thirty-two-year-old salesperson who has been working for a housewares company for three years. He has had rave reviews from customers and supervisors, and he feels that he deserves a raise. Dustin thinks that it is unfair that people less qualified, and who have worked at the company for less time than he has, have received raises. He has been afraid to ask for a raise for fear of appearing demanding and that he will be dismissed.

The Practice

The DEARMAN skill of DBT is a powerful way to improve your chance of getting more of what you want (Linehan 1993a, 1993b). DEARMAN is an acronym that stands for **D**escribe, **E**xpress, **A**ssert, **R**einforce, be **M**indful, **A**ct confident, and **N**egotiate. We have expanded on these ideas and come up with **DECREE**:

Define. Describe the situation by sticking to the facts. Don't add opinions or judgments. Dustin might say, "I've been working here for three years now and haven't received a raise. My performance reviews have always been positive, and my sales have increased every year." Saying something like "It's not fair that others are getting raises" is an opinion and judgment, and therefore is less of an effective approach.

Expect. Expect that things might not be easy, particularly if there has been a lot of conflict in the past. However, even if there is conflict don't compromise your values simply to keep a certain person in your life, or in Dustin's case just to keep the peace.

Communicate. Sit down with the person and communicate clearly about what it is that you want. State that you have spent some time thinking about the situation. Let him know exactly what it is that you are asking for.

Reinforce. It is a powerful intervention to get the other person to see what is in it for him to give you what you want. What you are doing is rewarding him for agreeing to your request. The idea is that if the other person does not gain from your request, he is less likely to agree. So Dustin might say, "I will be a lot happier and incentivized to work even harder if I get a salary that reflects my value to the company."

Express. Share your feelings about the situation. Use "I" statements without the expectation that the other person will be able to read your mind or know how you feel. Dustin might say, "Given how much I have put into my work and the results I have delivered, I believe that I deserve a raise."

Exhibit confidence. Many people have reasonable requests but act in ways that don't make them appear as if they deserve to get what they are asking for. Use a confident tone of voice, without whispering or stammering. Make reasonable eye contact. Stand up or sit up straight with your shoulders back and your chin up.

Here are more successful ways to go about asking for the things you want:

- **Stay flexible.** Your goal is to maintain a healthy relationship with other people. The idea is that there must be some give and take. Be prepared to negotiate and to offer and ask for alternative solutions. Dustin might agree to a smaller raise but with more vacation time or a greater contribution to his retirement fund. A helpful skill here is "turning the tables," which is the act of making the problem something for the other person to solve. So Dustin might say to his supervisor, "What do you think you can do?" or "I was thinking of a greater raise than 2 percent. I can't say yes to 2 percent, but I see that you consider me valuable, which I appreciate. What can we do here?"

- **Be firm.** If you have been a doormat and allowed people to trample over you in the past, the skill of standing up for yourself won't develop overnight. You have to practice letting go of the thoughts and emotions that led you to ineffective interactions in the past.

- **Have faith.** Believe in yourself. Know that you are as worthy as anyone else. Trust your instincts; there is wisdom within you. Don't let the opinions of others define you.

Checklist

☐ Have you defined the problem?

☐ Have you prepared for what could go wrong?

☐ Are you communicating clearly?

☐ Have you reinforced the other person?

☐ Are you exhibiting confidence?

☐ Are you ready to be flexible?

CHAPTER 5

Mood-Dependent Behavior

20 · Failing to Keep Commitments

The Problem

You make commitments that are important to you. You know that these engagements serve to maintain your goals and important relationships. But you have difficulty sticking to your commitments because your emotions are getting in the way. You may be 100 percent dedicated to meeting a friend for dinner, studying for an exam, or going to a meeting when you experience a strong emotion—say, sadness or anger—and then all of a sudden that commitment no longer feels important to you, and you do not follow through. You break your commitment.

When emotions impact your behavior, we refer to this as *mood-dependent behavior*. There are many problems with such behavior. First, you have made commitments that are important to you and your values; when you change them, you are likely moving away from important goals and values in your life. You can also be left with painful secondary emotions such as guilt, shame, regret, and even feelings of self-hatred and worthlessness when you realize you did not follow through on a commitment. Second, when commitments involve other people, you may be damaging important relationships by failing to keep them. Additionally, you may develop a reputation for not being reliable or trustworthy. Finally, you may be left feeling like you cannot trust yourself. You may worry that you will not be able to reach your goals, complete difficult tasks, or be in and keep relationships. When mood-dependent behavior happens repeatedly, you are left with powerful emotions and damaged relationships.

What It Looks Like

Thirty-seven-year-old Mei has had a particularly rough year. She has been struggling with balancing her career and family, caring for an elderly relative, and dealing with a particularly tense holiday season. A couple weeks ago Mei RSVP'd yes to a New Year's Eve party that she's excited about. She's looking forward to saying good-bye to the tough year and hello to a less-stressful future. Mei also made plans with a friend she hasn't seen in a while to go shopping for a dress, followed by dinner together, a few days before the party.

The shopping day starts out fine. Mei has a nice breakfast then goes for a run, thinking about how the mall will be a nice change of pace from an ordinary Saturday. But when she gets home, she becomes infuriated by her still-sleeping husband. He is always on her case for sleeping the day away, and now he is the one on the verge of being late for work. Her anger begins to rise as she goes to wake him up. The fight starts quickly, and they both begin yelling and saying hurtful things to each other. Mei goes into another room and begins crying. She is consumed with anger, sadness, and now the secondary emotion of fear that her marriage will end. She crawls into bed feeling guilty about her anger and utterly hopeless. She can't imagine going to the mall and no longer cares about the party. She texts her friend to say that she is sick and can't go shopping. Then Mei goes online and changes her RSVP to "not coming" and stays in her house for the rest of the weekend.

The Practice

Here is how you address the difficulty of keeping important commitments:

- **Be mindful of your current emotion.** Step back and pay attention to all the ways that you are feeling (Linehan 1993a, 1993b). Often situations prompt multiple emotions that can get tangled up in your mind, leaving you feeling bad. Find a quiet space and take a few deep breaths. Ask yourself what emotions you are feeling. Look for clues in your body. Are you crying? Are your muscles tense? Are you crossing your arms or clenching your fists? Notice any urges you have. Do you want to avoid people or crawl into bed? Do you want to yell or throw something? Your body and urges will give you clues. Before reacting, name the emotion or emotions that you are feeling. Stay with naming the emotions. Do not act on any of the urges, just notice and label (nonjudgmentally) what you are feeling. Stick to the facts.

- **Identify what you were feeling before.** When your emotions change, it can be difficult to remember what you were thinking and feeling before something prompted an intense emotion. Now that you have been mindful of your current emotions, step back and ask yourself: what was I feeling before my emotions became so intense? Sit quietly, take some deep breaths, and think about what prompted your intense emotions and what was happening before that prompt. For example, Mei's feelings of intense anger were prompted when she saw that her husband was still sleeping. Prior to that she was not angry at all; in fact, she was content and looking forward to meeting a friend and going to the mall.

    If you are having difficulty, retrace your steps. Start with the beginning of the day, or even the night before, and identify the chain of events, thoughts, and feelings to help you figure out what prompted your emotions and how you felt before and after. In DBT, this is called a chain analysis (Linehan 1993a, 1993b).

- **Think dialectically and validate both.** Thinking *dialectically*, or holding two seemingly opposing things in your mind at once, is a core DBT skill (Linehan 1993a, 1993b). It is very challenging to do, but it can help you see the complexity of the situation as a whole. Once you have identified what prompted your intense emotions, and how you were feeling before and after that prompt, your task is to validate both experiences, even if they are completely opposite.

Remember: you must find what makes sense about each experience—that is where you'll find the wisdom in the moment. Stay away from using "should" or "shouldn't"— really look for what makes sense about how you feel. For example, it makes sense that Mei was excited to go to the mall and see a friend, angry when she noticed her husband sleeping, and guilty about how she woke him up. All are true. Remember to validate feelings and *not* behaviors. Mei's feelings of anger make sense; however, the way she addressed those feelings may have been ineffective. Validating feelings can also help you change behaviors and repair relationships.

- **Remember your long-term goals.** Often when you break commitments, you are making a decision based on how you feel in the moment. As a result, you are not attending to your long-term goals. For some people, those goals go completely out of their minds. Once you have been able to think dialectically and validate your entire and often conflicting emotional experience, step back and identify your long-term goals. Try thinking about your relationship goals as well as goals to attend or complete specific tasks. Sometimes keeping a list of long-term goals in a journal can be useful so that you can refer to them when you notice urges to change your commitments.

- **Wait a few hours before breaking your commitments.** If possible, try giving yourself two to twenty-four hours before changing your commitments or goals. Avoid reacting immediately to how you feel in the moment. In this example, Mei may not have been able to wait to decide about her commitment to go to the mall, but she certainly could have waited before changing her RSVP to the party or canceling her dinner plans.

Slowing down and pausing before breaking plans gives you time to self-validate, use DBT skills, and see if the intensity of your emotions decreases. When your emotions are intense, it is very challenging to think through your options. This is because in times when your emotions are greatest, areas of the brain that help you think and reason are less active. In an effort to preserve your long-term goals, give your emotions time to become less intense; then you can think through the pros and cons of changing commitments that were at one time important to you.

Checklist

☐ Have you validated your emotions?

☐ Have you identified your long-term goals?

☐ Have you waited at least two hours before making any decisions that may have long-term consequences?

21 • QUITTING WORK OR SCHOOL

The Problem

You are feeling miserable and unappreciated. All you want to do is lie in bed and not deal with the world. You have school or work obligations, but your urge is to not go. You have half an hour to rise, shower, get dressed, and leave the house—the whole endeavor feels overwhelming.

What It Looks Like

Nineteen-year-old Heather has been working for six weeks as a barista at her local coffee shop, and she's proud that she has lasted this long. Everything is going well. If she can do another six weeks, she will get a small pay raise and qualify for health insurance and the retirement plan. All her previous jobs had lasted only a few days and ended with her quitting. She likes her current coworkers and customers, and the pace of the work keeps her busy enough to distract her from the annoyances of her daily life. Last night, though, she had a fight with her boyfriend and now feels that it marks the end of everything. She notices that she is having catastrophizing thoughts that overwhelm her and make her feel miserable. Even though she had a good night's sleep, she wants to give up and stay in bed.

Quitting work or school has consequences. It will harm your reputation, and it will make it hard to get a job, as it will be nearly impossible to get references. You will be known by others as a quitter. If staying in school is difficult and quitting seems like the best solution, know that finding a satisfying job without a degree will be *much* more difficult. If you are quitting a job out of retaliation, remember that most jobs can be easily filled by someone else; even if your leaving is a temporary inconvenience for your workplace, you will quickly be forgotten when someone else steps into the position. You will not have made your point—worse, you will be left jobless. Moreover, if you established a friendship with your coworkers, these relationships will suffer not only because of your unreliability but also because they will need to pick up your shifts once you leave. Finally, if you have been relying on the job for money and benefits, you will lose all of this as well.

The Practice

Here is how to combat the tendency to want to quit a job, school, or some other major commitment:

- **Notice that you are stuck.** The first step is to recognize that you feel at a loss for what to do next. One useful trick is to change your perspective; instead of saying to yourself "I am stuck," use your own name. In the example above, Heather might say, "Heather, you are stuck and you are struggling to get out of bed and go off to work." The act of using your own name allows you to become your own friendly advisor.

- **Un-pair unrelated situations.** Perhaps you are upset because of a fight with your parent, or because it rained while you were on your beach vacation. You can always validate that it makes sense that you are upset; however, neither the rain nor the argument with Dad has anything to do with whether you should quit work or school. Heather would say something like "I am really upset by what happened last night with my boyfriend. However, that has nothing to do with my job."

- **Consider your values.** If the reason why you don't want to go to work or school *is* related to those places—perhaps you had a fight with your boss or coworker, or professor or fellow student—then you need to determine whether what happened is something that goes against your personal values or left you feeling shame. For example, if you have been reprimanded by your boss for consistently showing up late, you might feel shame or guilt. You should then work on taking the feedback to heart and coming up with a plan to correct your tardiness. Alternatively, if your boss asked you on a date in order for you to get better work shifts, you might seriously consider whether you want to work at a place that condones such behavior.

- **Review your long-term goals.** Remind yourself why you have your job in the first place and how it fits into your life plan. Decide whether not going to work is consistent with this goal. For Heather, the pride of being able to hold down her job and proving to herself and others that she can do this is consistent with her long-term goals.

- **Make a pros and cons list.** Identify all the pros and cons of going to work *and* the pros and cons of not going to work (Linehan 1993a, 1993b).

- **Act opposite to your action urge.** If you have come to the conclusion that not going to work or school is based on your current mood and not consistent with your long-term plan, then act opposite to your urge. If you have an intense desire to stay in bed, instead get up and go! Your current emotional state will pass.

Checklist

- ☐ Have you paid attention to your being stuck?
- ☐ Have you un-paired unrelated situations?
- ☐ If your situations are related, have you considered your value system?
- ☐ Is quitting consistent with your goals?
- ☐ Can you use an opposite action to fight the urge to quit?

22 · Feeling Like Skills Are Not Working

The Problem

You have been trying to deal with a difficult situation and are ready to give up because nothing seems to help. Strong emotions kill your motivation, and it takes a huge effort to do almost anything. It seems that nothing is working out. No matter how hard you try, everything just seems to collapse. All the skills you have learned, including those that have worked before, don't seem to be working now.

What It Looks Like

After twenty-eight-year-old Jason broke up with his girlfriend, he felt that his entire world was collapsing. He had gone for more than a year without using drugs or being self-injurious. Jason felt that he was on his way to recovery. But when his girlfriend left, he called himself a "bag of emotions." He tries going for walks, cleaning his room, breathing deeply, and distracting himself, but his mind keeps going back to how terrible he is feeling without her. He also keeps thinking about how all the skills he is trying do not help.

The Practice

Feeling like nothing is going to help is a common experience for people with BPD. The mnemonic **CAn DO IT** is helpful for remembering the steps to take to end the feeling that nothing can help. The following *will* help:

1. Commit to persist. When nothing is working out, it is easy to want to stay in bed, quit, or go back to self-destructive behaviors like drug use or self-injury. Doing something—anything—other than these maladaptive behaviors is a victory, even if you feel it is not. Make a commitment to keep on trying; the longer you stay fighting, the better the chance of victory.

2. Acknowledge self-validation. Acknowledge just how hard this is. Remember that the feelings that come up when you are in this kind of distress make sense. Ask yourself if you have forgotten to validate your experience. Are you trying too hard or trying to do too much in spite of how you are feeling? The result of not feeling any success can lead to even more frustration. Slow things down, take a deep breath. Acknowledge what you are feeling and that you are trying.

3. Define your goal. Rather than staying miserable and defeated, ask yourself, "What is my goal? Is what I am doing helping me reach my goal?" When skills don't work, it is generally because of one of two reasons. The first reason is that you haven't defined the actual problem. For instance, if you are angry with your mother because you are sad that your friend didn't keep a dinner date, the problem is that you are sad about the date situation. Fighting with your mother in response to that emotion is not the solution and likely creates other problems. Defining the problem would be saying, "I am sad that my friend did not keep the date." The solution would be to address your relationship with your friend, or mourn the loss of the friendship if the friendship is ending. The second reason new behaviors might not work is that you are using the wrong approach to a problem you have defined. For instance, going for a long run, which might make you feel good under other circumstances, won't help if you are already exhausted.

So the first thing to do is clearly define the goal. In the example, Jason wanted to stop thinking about his ex. Yet, when he cleaned his room he saw all the clothes that she had bought him, and this caused his intense emotions to return. In this situation, cleaning his room wasn't helping him suffer less, and it wasn't moving him toward his goal.

4. **O**pen yourself to one thing in the moment (Linehan 1993a, 1993b). Now that you have defined your goal, you will realize that in many cases it is impossible to solve the problem with one action. So try several different solutions if you must, but only practice one at a time. If the first solution does not work, move on to your next idea and then do only that one in the moment. Experience the success of each task that brings you closer to your goal.

5. **I**nitiate generosity. Getting overly self-focused or self-absorbed can be a natural consequence of high levels of emotional distress. It is important to turn your attention away from yourself and to do something kind and compassionate for someone else, someone you care about. When you do something kind for someone else, your mood will lift and you will also find compassion for yourself.

6. **T**hank life. All of the frustrations and obstacles in life are opportunities to practice a more effective and skillful way of living, even if you don't feel like that in the moment. If you can find it within yourself, thank life for giving you an opportunity to practice dealing with difficult moments. This may be the most difficult practice, because thinking of gratitude when you are suffering seems impossible. Be gentle as you practice. In time you will see that life prepares you for all kinds of difficult tasks, each of which can be an opportunity to practice mastery. If you can celebrate the difficult moments as a gift, they will begin to lose their painful power over your emotional state.

Checklist

☐ Did you catch your thought that skills don't work?

☐ Have you recognized that you are close to giving up?

☐ Have you practiced CAn DO IT?

CHAPTER 6

Feeling Unreal

23 · WHEN YOU DON'T FEEL REAL

The Problem

You have the occasional experience, especially when you are under stress, that you are not real, that you exist outside of your body. The problem is that it is hard to know who you are and what your experience is. Being in relationships with others, and participating in various activities, can feel overly complicated, particularly when you don't know what is you and what is not you.

What It Looks Like

Georgina is a twenty-four-year-old with BPD who experienced sexual abuse by an uncle when she was between the ages of five and eight. She comes into therapy and says, "The other day, as I headed to work, I suddenly found myself looking through the window of my office at myself. I've had out-of-body experiences before, but this was the weirdest one I've ever had. For the past sixteen years, I have never completely felt that I was in my body, and this time I felt totally spaced out."

This experience of not feeling real is called *depersonalization*. It happens when your emotions are so powerful that you disconnect from experiencing them. Depersonalization can include the sensation that you're an outside observer of your thoughts, emotions, and body or parts of your body. You might experience a sense of floating above yourself or that you are dreaming. People who experience depersonalization sometimes say that they are not in control of what they do or what they say. You might feel as if your face, body, and limbs are distorted. Emotionally, you might feel numb or that the things that you remember about your past have no emotions connected to them.

It is difficult to make and keep relationships with people or go about the business of your life when you are not connected to it.

The Practice

The first thing to do is notice that you are disconnecting. It is essential that you know what your disconnection experience is. Perhaps it is that you don't feel your body, or maybe that your thoughts are not your own. It is important to know what specifically happens to you when you are experiencing depersonalization.

The quickest way to get out of a depersonalized state is to get grounded. Most times you ought to be able to get grounded before depersonalization gets too bad. *Grounding* is the skill of connecting yourself to your emotions and experiences. The most effective way to get grounded is to do something that will keep you in the present moment. The ultimate task is to be able to experience situations that would typically elicit depersonalization without depersonalizing. Grounding techniques typically involve participation in a neutral activity that will not cause emotional pain and will keep the person present.

- **Try a grounding technique.** When you notice depersonalization coming on, label the present moment in terms of day, date, and place. You might say, "Today is Thursday, February 19." You can also tell yourself what you are doing in the present moment, such as "I am doing laundry" or "I am having a cup of tea."

  If you are continuing to slip into the depersonalized state, then select some category and then name items within that category. For instance, if the category you choose is "blue items in the room," you would then look around the room and name everything in the room that is the color blue. Or if your category is animals, you could choose to name every animal you know from A to Z.

A third technique to try is balancing on one leg. It is difficult for a person to balance *and* experience depersonalization, so you can always stop what you're doing and strike a one-legged pose.

- **Focus on using your senses.** Perhaps the quickest way to get present is through strong physical sensation (Linehan 1993a, 1993b), like focusing on cold by holding an ice cube, or focusing on a strong fragrance by using a strong-smelling balm, or concentrating on taste by sucking on a flavorful mint. Consider carrying a box of mints in your pocket or purse if you are going to be in a situation that has historically triggered depersonalization and where doing something like balancing might look awkward.

- **Ask for help.** If the depersonalization is too powerful, you may not be able to ground yourself alone. Having someone who knows this about you can mean that she can help at that time.

Checklist

☐ Did you notice early indications that you are beginning to disconnect?

☐ Can you name the place, date, and activity you are doing?

☐ Can you name items in a category?

☐ Have you tried standing on one leg or sucking on a powerful mint?

☐ Have you reached out to a support person?

24 · When the World Does Not Seem Real

The Problem

Related to the problem of not feeling real is the problem of feeling that the rest of the world does not feel real—although you feel real. The sensation is that you are living in an alien environment. Another name for this experience is *derealization.*

What It Looks Like

Graham is a thirty-two-year-old man with BPD. He was sexually abused as a child by a neighbor. In recent years, when he has been visiting his parents, he's noticed that being back in his childhood neighborhood triggers the feeling that the world is not real. It is a sensation he describes as watching the world go on around him from the seats of a movie theater, as if the events around him are scenes from a film. He feels as if he is able to see what goes on about him but can't participate in the events.

The Practice

Similar to the skills recommended to combat depersonalization (see situation 23, "When You Don't Feel Real"), the goal is to get grounded. Here are some other techniques you can use to ground yourself when you experience the world as not being real:

- **Be observant.** Keep your eyes open, look around the space you are in, notice details, and list facts about your surroundings.

- **Change the temperature.** Place a cool, damp cloth over your face, or hold something cool such as a pack of frozen peas.

- **Use five present-moment questions.** Ask yourself, and then answer: "Where am I? How old am I? What am I wearing? What season is it? What is my telephone number?"

- **Listen carefully.** Focus on a neutral sound, like the chirping of a bird or the hum of an air conditioner.

Checklist

☐ Are you keeping your eyes open?

☐ Can you name and label items in your environment?

☐ Have you asked yourself five present-moment questions?

☐ Can you focus on a neutral sound?

CHAPTER 7

Who Am I?

25 · Not Knowing How to Act

The Problem

You may have noticed that you are struggling with a sense of knowing who you are, and that because of this you are struggling with knowing how to behave. You might change the way you dress and speak—you might even change the values or social norms that you uphold—depending on how the people around you behave. Your feelings are more than simply a desire to fit in; it's a real struggle knowing who you are and how you want to behave around other people and in different situations. Not knowing how to act makes even the most typical interpersonal situations very anxiety provoking.

What It Looks Like

Twenty-three-year-old Clara has difficulty maintaining relationships. She is often hopelessly lonely and cannot seem to feel connected or like she belongs with any group of people. She has had this problem since she was really young. In high school she changed social groups often, starting out grunge, then emo. Then she started running and was considered sporty, and finally she ended high school more preppy. This pattern continued throughout college. Now as an adult her changes are subtler, but she cannot seem to figure out how to act when she is around people she wants to be friends with. She notices more and more anxiety before social engagements.

A new friend that she met at a dinner party invited Clara to hang out with a bunch of her friends. Clara accepted the invitation, and later she called her friend to see what was planned for the evening. She learned that they would be going with a big group of people to a bar and then a metal concert. Clara doesn't like metal, and she's been to that bar once or twice and found it dirty with much of its staff demeaning to women. Nevertheless, she pulls out an old metal band T-shirt and goes to meet the group. After an hour or so, Clara's friend pulls her aside and asks if everything is okay. Clara looks confused. Her friend says that she has never seen her like this, swearing often and acting cool and dismissive. Clara says, "This is who I am when I'm having fun." Clara turns her back to her friend and keeps talking to two guys. Her friend doesn't call her to hang out again.

The Practice

Many people with BPD find that they morph, acting differently depending on whom they are around. Sometimes these people are referred to as social chameleons. Here is how you address the feeling of not knowing how to act:

- **Identify your values.** Part of beginning to know who you are and how to act is identifying and paying attention to your values. Your values are the guiding principles you live by. They help you navigate life. They are whatever standards you feel are important. Many people do not spend time explicitly thinking about their values; however, your values will help you figure out how to act and what to prioritize. And when you have clear recognition of your values, it becomes easier to see when your behavior would cross your values, since going against your values frequently leads to feelings of guilt and shame.

- **Identify your goals.** Like identifying your values, identifying your goals will help you know how to act. Consider both long- and short-term goals that you have for relationships as well as your life. When you are not sure how to act, ask yourself, "What is my goal?" Then consider if your behavior matches up with that goal. For example, Clara's goal is to make some new friends; however, in the process she lost the very friend that invited her out. In addition, Clara violated her values around speaking respectfully to those she cares about by taking on the style of communication of the group that she assumed included swearing and being disrespectful.

- **Ground yourself.** When you are anxious or swept up in social situations, the urge to take on other people's behavior can be very intense. You must ground yourself so that you can connect with your own values and goals. Try these grounding practices for a few minutes as soon as you feel the urge to act differently:

  Identify everything in the room that is a certain color. Go through the five senses in a similar way, such as identifying all the sounds you can hear.

  Pick a category and identify one thing from that category that begins with each letter of the alphabet. For example, name all the fruits and vegetables you can think of from A to Z.

  Eat a sour or spicy candy and mindfully pay attention to the sensations in your mouth. It's helpful to keep a tin of candy in your purse or pocket for this purpose.

  Once you are grounded, review your goals and values. Ask yourself, "How do I need to act in order to behave according to my values and in line with my goals?" Be mindful that these are *your* values and that you are not temporarily taking on other people's values in order to fit in or be accepted.

- **Plan ahead.** When you are practicing new skills it can be very useful to make a plan, also known as the DBT skill *cope ahead* (Linehan 1993a, 1993b). When you notice anxiety about how to act, make a plan. On a piece of paper, write out your goals for the interaction and any long-term social goals that you have. Next, write down your values about how you want to behave and how you want to treat people and be treated. Write out a plan of ways that you can act according to your goals and values. Next, identify the barriers to your skillful plan. What are common pitfalls that may show up? For example, anticipate pressure you may feel to fit in and think about what behaviors you may engage in that cross your values or go against your goals. Make a commitment to stick to your plan.

Checklist

☐ Have you identified your values?

☐ Have you identified short- and long-term goals?

☐ Have you made a plan for how to cope in the future?

The Problem

You may have noticed that you are very sensitive to other people's emotions. You may feel as if you are porous—like an emotional sponge. You may have been told that you are very empathetic, or you may have been called an empath. You notice your own feelings of sadness when you are with a friend who has had a loss, or of anger when a family member is recounting a story that makes him angry. Being able to feel other people's emotions can be a wonderful thing and mean that people feel understood by you; however, when you take on others' emotions without awareness, it causes you a lot of suffering.

What It Looks Like

Carrie is forty years old and prides herself on being a supportive friend. While on the phone, Carrie listens to her distraught best friend reminisce about her mom, who had recently passed away. Carrie can feel her friend's pain deep in her own chest; Carrie even cries while on the phone. After the call, Carrie crawls into bed. She notices waves of fear and feelings of loss. As she notices the feelings, she starts thinking about why. She begins thinking about losing people in her life and having to live alone. Sadness envelops her. She is so overwhelmed by fear and sorrow that Carrie feels almost unable to move. This sadness continues for the next few days. Carrie can't understand what is happening, as lately her mood has been steady and she has been experiencing a lot of joy and accomplishing many goals.

The Practice

Here is how you can avoid taking on the feelings and emotions of others unnecessarily:

- **Notice the change in your emotional state.** If you know that you are going to be spending time with someone who is experiencing strong emotions, check in with yourself first; notice and label your emotions before you connect with the other person. It may be useful to write your emotions down. Once you are with that person and the strong emotions arise, be mindful of how your experience changes. When you are no longer with the person, pay attention to how you feel. Label your emotions and ask yourself how you were feeling before you met with the person. Notice the change in your emotional experience.

- **Identify which emotions belong to you.** Once you have noticed the change, ask yourself, "Which emotions belong to me?" When you take on others' emotions you may end up trying to validate how you are feeling by finding examples in your life to confirm those feelings, even if they are not relevant to the present. For example, Carrie took on her friend's feelings of sadness and loss, and instead of noticing sadness for her friend, she took on the friend's feelings, which created thoughts about loss in her own life, which quickly consumed her. Taking on other people's intense emotions influences your thinking; your mind begins to come up with examples from your own life that validate the very emotions that do not belong to you.

- **Let others have their emotions.** Letting other people have their own emotions can be challenging when you are not aware whose emotions belong to whom. Now that you are aware of your feelings and your friend's you can validate both. Ask yourself, "What am I feeling?" Then ask yourself, "What is she feeling?" Practice using phrases like "I am

103

feeling _____ . And when _____ happened I started feeling _____." Articulate what you are feeling and what the other person is feeling or doing. Do your best to keep the experiences separate. Then you can see the wisdom in both emotional experiences. You may have feelings about the other person's experience, which you should articulate. In the example above, Carrie might say, "I am feeling sadness for my friend's loss." Notice that you are not simply saying "I am feeling sadness"—work on really making your experience separate and unique.

- **Plan ahead for emotionally intense interpersonal situations.** Make a plan to help yourself not get emotionally confused in these situations. Practice being mindful of your current emotion before, during, and after these interactions. Then develop a strategy to self-soothe afterward, to help you return to your emotional baseline.

Checklist

☐ Have you identified what you felt before the interaction?

☐ Have you asked yourself what emotions belong to the other person?

☐ Have you identified three ways to self-soothe once you have left the interaction?

27 · Constantly Changing Who You Are

The Problem

You are trying to connect with a group of people. Rather than being yourself, you change your behavior to fit in with them. The problem is that when you are at work you act one way, when you are at home you act another way, and when you are with friends you act yet another way. It becomes particularly difficult when your various groups overlap. You keep changing because you want to be accepted; however, this behavior doesn't help you develop your own identity.

What It Looks Like

Susannah is a thirty-three-year-old office administrator who struggles with self-acceptance, although outwardly she seems to be well liked. She acts quiet and shy at work, confident and flirtatious at her gym, subdued and withdrawn with her family, and easygoing and adventurous with friends. Susannah is a social chameleon, which works when she is with any one group, but she is terrified that one day her various groups will bump into each other and discover that she is a fraud—and she's afraid that she won't know how to act. She wishes she could be herself but is not sure who that is.

Like Susannah, most of us want to make a good impression, but for some people with BPD this desire is based on a desperate need for acceptance rather than on simple social pleasantries. For you, being a social chameleon and striving to fit in can come at a huge psychological cost, because you continually have to monitor your social performance—when your behavior or attitude doesn't appear to be having the desired effect, you feel like you have to keep adjusting yourself. You may be aware of paying very careful attention to others' behavior, so that you know what is expected before you make a response. Or you may notice behaving as you imagine others want you to behave, or trying to get people who might not like you to like you.

It turns out that people who are really good at making great impressions tend to have less-stable intimate relationships because of this constantly changing behavior (Snyder 1974). On the other hand, being too rigid in how you act isn't the way to fit in either; a person whose sense of self is overly strong and not flexible suffers a social cost as well.

The Practice

Being flexible in different environments and social situations is a great quality. But it's important to strive for balance: Being overly flexible to the point where you are always changing is not healthy, nor is being so inflexible that you can't tolerate anything outside your comfort zone. This extreme behavior comes at the cost of being who you are. Here are ways to help yourself:

- **Define your values.** In order to be yourself, you have to stick to your values. And to do that, you first have to know what your values are. Defining your values will allow you to feel confident enough to go with what feels right for you. This way, you won't need to always be looking to others to feel good about your choices, thoughts, and behaviors.

  Keep a values journal in which you record on a regular basis the things that make you proud: the choices you've made, the times you have stayed true to your core beliefs, and the things that feel right to you even when no one is around. Your personal values list might include integrity, honesty, compassion, achievement, accountability, effectiveness, generosity, and so on.

- **Let go of seeking approval and reassurance from others.** Once you have established your values, pay attention to when you are looking for the approval of others. Then practice letting go of seeking reassurance from others. You need to approve your own behavior. In order to do this you have to pay attention to how you talk, think, and behave when you are with your various groups. Notice when your behavior comes mainly from wanting someone else to say that you fit in or that you did the right thing. Before deciding what action to take in any given situation, check in with yourself to see if your choice is consistent with your values.

- **Notice if your commitments are consistent with your goals.** Finally, before you take on a new commitment—like applying for a new job, starting college, or beginning a new romantic relationship—you must examine whether you are doing this because it is the right action for you, based on your values, or whether you are doing this because you want approval from others. If you have doubts, go back to your values journal. If what you are doing is simply or mainly for others, continue to work on reducing this behavior and increasing the behavior of doing the things that you have defined as your core self.

Checklist

☐ Are you doing things mainly for others?

☐ Have you started a values journal?

☐ Have you practiced letting go of approval seeking?

☐ Are your commitments consistent with your goals?

CHAPTER 8

Procrastination

28 · NOT COMPLETING A PROJECT

The Problem

Completing a project can be a daunting task. Sometimes a project feels so overwhelming that it seems impossible to do, and the only option that comes to mind is to abandon it despite the negative consequences. You know you need to get the project done but it just feels impossible. You feel doomed.

What It Looks Like

Eighteen-year-old Rocco is a freshman in college. He often struggled to get homework done in high school, but his mother had always helped him complete things at the last minute. Rocco had been meaning to start the project he was recently assigned a week ago, but each time he sat down to write, his heart would begin to pound and his anxiety would rise. "I can't do it!" he would say, then quickly abandon the project for other things. Now, the night before the project is due, Rocco wants to jump out of his skin. He stares at a blank screen for a few minutes and then gets up from his computer. His mind is filled with thoughts of being stupid and that he can't do this project; the certainty of failure looms large. Doing well in school is important to Rocco, and he knows that he will feel like a complete failure if he doesn't complete the project. As Rocco's anxiety and feelings of worthlessness increase, so do his urges to engage in self-destructive behaviors.

The Practice

Here is how you address the type of procrastination associated with not completing a project or task:

- **Self-validate and let go of your judgments.** Doing projects is hard, so it is important that you acknowledge that. Moreover, it is much more difficult to get things done when you judge yourself. Acknowledge the challenge you're facing and your anxiety, stick to the facts, and let go of your judgments.

- **Give yourself encouragement.** Replace "I can't" with some words of encouragement that will help you complete your project. You can use statements like "I can do this" or "I will feel accomplished and a sense of mastery when I am finished." You can write these statements on a sticky note and then place it on or near your computer so that you can see it while you are working. Telling yourself that you can do something can lead to a self-fulfilling prophecy of success.

- **Make a plan and reward yourself.** Getting started on your project can be the hardest part. So take baby steps, first by making a rough outline of your project. Use bullet points for the major elements of your project. Then break down those points by writing some supporting ideas. Next, make a plan about which elements or sections you will complete first— and when you will take a break. At each break, give yourself a small reward for completing that task. Consider using rewards like checking your e-mail, watching fifteen to thirty minutes of TV, having a snack, going for a walk or run, or calling a friend to talk briefly. Pick something that will motivate you to finish each part of the project.

- **Say no to social media or e-mail.** Save checking social media, e-mail, online news sites, or shopping until one of your breaks. Tell yourself, "I cannot go online until I have finished a section or finished my project." Going online is a great distraction and just another way to procrastinate!

- **Review your long-term goals.** Remembering your long-term goals can be very helpful and motivating when you have the urge to procrastinate. Play out in your mind the situation of not doing the project. What will it feel like to go to class or work and not turn in the project? What thoughts and feelings will you have? What will it be like to get a failing grade or poor performance review? How will not doing this project impact your anxiety when your next project is due?

- **Complete a pros and cons list.** Write out a pros and cons list on a piece of paper to look at all of your options. Make a list of the pros of finishing the project and the cons of finishing the project, as well as the pros of not finishing the project and the cons of not finishing the project. Next, go back to your list and circle all the long-term pros and long-term cons on each list. It is important to look not just at the number of pros and cons but whether they have a long-term positive or negative impact on your life.

Checklist

☐   Did you validate your anxiety and fear of failure?

☐   Have you recognized ways you are avoiding the project?

☐   Have you encouraged yourself?

☐   Did you review your long-term goals?

☐   Have you completed a pros and cons list?

29 · NOT COMPLETING AN APPLICATION

The Problem

You are struggling to complete a job application form. At first you feel anxious, then afraid. Because of this fear you don't even start the process, even though it is in your long-term interest to complete the form.

What It Looks Like

Abbie is twenty-one years old and has wanted to get a job since high school, but each time she is faced with an application she is filled with panic and self-loathing. Abbie worries that she is not skilled enough or that people will think she is stupid and unqualified. Her catastrophizing thoughts become an emotional roller coaster that leads to the conclusion that she will be unwanted, so applying becomes pointless. Despite being qualified for many jobs, Abbie now lacks confidence and typically gives up before even requesting an application. Abbie wonders what people will think about a twenty-one-year-old who has never worked. As time passes and Abbie continues to avoid job applications, she fears that she will go nowhere in life, which sometimes leads her to think that her life is pointless. This makes each opportunity to apply for a job more difficult.

The Practice

Here is how you address the type of procrastination and anxiety that come with filling out a job application:

- **Self-validate.** The thought of filling out a job application can bring up feelings of anxiety, uncertainty about your skills and abilities, worries about being judged, fears of failure and not being good enough, and fears about your future. By self-validating, or acknowledging your feelings, you can identify some of the barriers that are causing you to procrastinate. Then you can use your skills to decrease the intensity of the difficult thoughts and feelings. It is also a time to let go of your judgments and be kind to yourself. Ask yourself, "Would I understand if one of my friends felt this way about completing this application? What would I tell her?" Be mindful to not judge yourself for procrastinating. We all put things off; the key is to get back on track and face both your own anxiety and the task of completing your application.

- **Make a pros and cons list.** What are the long-term consequences of completing your application? What are the long-term consequences of avoiding this application? Write down the pros and cons of each action. Notice if this type of procrastination is a pattern for you and if it has had negative consequences in your life. Ask yourself, "Do I want to have that experience again?" Be mindful that, in the moment, the short-term pros of avoiding the application can feel very powerful; however, procrastination is a very short-term cure for your anxiety.

- **Focus on what is in it for you.** Sometimes when you are faced with challenging experiences and painful feelings, it can help to focus on any benefits you will gain from going through the experience, even when it is painful. Can you make meaning out of the experience? One thing to consider is whether doing this hard task will leave you with a sense of mastery or independence.

- **Ask for help.** Sometimes you just need help, and asking for assistance is a good start. Some people have difficulty asking for help, but keep in mind that nearly every adult has had to complete applications, so finding someone with experience shouldn't be one of your worries. Ask someone who you think could help you think through what to write or even sit with you as you begin the application. Consider family, friends, teachers, mentors, colleagues, or someone you know in a similar field of study or career type. You may just need someone who helps calm you down when you feel anxious or who is a good cheerleader and will help you stay motivated. Some people judge themselves for not being able to complete an application on their own; let that judgment go. Asking for help is a great skill to practice and one that you will use for the rest of your life.

Checklist

☐ Have you self-validated?

☐ Have you reminded yourself why you want to complete this application?

☐ Have you identified people who could help you?

30 · Skipping Work or Class

The Problem

When you are having a difficult time, you might occasionally skip work, class, or other obligations—even though it goes against your values. For some, skipping commitments is a chronic problem that has serious results: job loss, failing grades, and so on. This behavior is extremely common for people who struggle to regulate their emotions.

What It Looks Like

Cara is a bright and articulate thirty-year-old woman with a degree in education. She loves working with children and has wanted to be a teacher since she was young. She struggles to manage her emotions, which often get the best of her, leading her to change her goals and priorities when she feels her emotions intensely. Last night, Cara and her boyfriend got into a fight, and he threatened to break up with her. Hoping wine would solve her problems, she had a few drinks and went to bed. Now her alarm is going off, and she doesn't want to get out of bed. Cara can't stop thinking about their fight and how angry and sad she is. She feels hungover and empty.

These fights happen often, and they usually take a couple of days to resolve. She knows that she needs to go to work, but nothing seems to matter anymore. Cara has been fired from four different teaching jobs in the last two years for coming in late or not showing up. She is beginning to worry that the next time she gets fired she won't be able to find another job. But feeling dreadful on this morning, Cara rolls over and goes back to sleep.

The Practice

Here is how you address the behavior of skipping class, work, or other commitments:

- **Plan ahead.** If your emotions get in the way of getting to or staying at work, school, or another major obligation, you need a plan. Identify what emotions lead to the urge to skip commitments—perhaps sadness, fear, shame, or guilt. Make a plan for how you will decrease the intensity of the emotions that lead you to avoidant behavior. Consider acting opposite to the urge to avoid. Most people experience a positive change in their emotional state when they get to work, school, or whatever the destination.

- **Remember that emotions change.** Remind yourself that painful emotions change. Sometimes you will feel stuck, and it might feel like your pain will never end. Remember that all emotions change, especially if you pay attention to them (even the painful ones!). Sit in a quiet space or even outside, and bring your attention to your breath. Notice your inhale and exhale. When your mind wanders to other thoughts or feelings, gently turn your attention back to your inhale and exhale. If you have difficulty just sitting, take a mindful walk and focus on your breath or your natural surroundings. Notice how you feel after ten minutes. Try to relax your body.

- **Postpone the decision.** Instead of telling yourself that you will not go, allow yourself to put off the decision for fifteen or so minutes. In DBT, this skill is known as *adaptive denial* (Linehan 2014a, 2014b). Even if you feel strongly that you can't or won't go, get dressed and ready anyway. You can always get undressed and back into bed later! Take a shower or wash up, get dressed, and do anything else to make yourself ready. Once you have done all these steps and the fifteen minutes have passed, reevaluate and see if you feel differently about skipping.

- **Check in with someone to stay accountable.** Ask someone in your life to check in with you before you have to go to work, school, a meeting, or some other regular commitment. You may find it easier to not fall into skipping behavior if you are directly accountable to someone in your life. Try to set up a schedule of checking in or texting someone to let her know that you're on your way to work, school, or an appointment. Ask her to check in with you, if she doesn't hear from you.

- **Avoid mood-altering substances.** Mood-altering substances can worsen mood-dependent behavior, especially in people who struggle with BPD or have difficulty regulating their emotions. If you have a pattern of skipping work, school, or other commitments, do an experiment: for one week do not use any mood-altering substances and notice if your skipping behavior decreases.

Checklist

☐   Have you reviewed your plan for how to cope?

☐   Have you checked in with someone to whom you feel accountable?

☐   Are you out of bed and dressed?

31 · NOT GETTING OUT OF BED

The Problem

You may find that there are times when you wake up in the morning and life feels so overwhelming that you cannot imagine getting out of bed. At your worst, staying in bed can feel like the only option. Staying in bed may help you avoid difficult and possibly painful situations, but it can also result in missing work or school, breaking plans with people you care about, and not following through on important commitments. Staying in bed is a short-term solution that can lead to many of the common problems that come from avoiding life's tasks or obligations based on your mood.

What It Looks Like

Ethan is twenty-six years old and finds both his part-time job and night school very stressful. Today he has both a midterm assignment due and a shift at work with a manager he doesn't like. His mood has been low for the last week, and he stayed up late watching TV every night, too stressed to study. "I'm going to fail anyway," he told himself. As his morning alarm continues to beep, he feels like he will fail his test and that he should quit his job because his manager hates him anyway. He starts to think about what to do. Ethan knows that the effective thing to do is to get up, because missing the exam and work will be stressful and lead to more feelings of failure and fear that he will get fired. He also knows that staying in bed all day feels good for a few hours, then he begins to feel worthless and like a failure. He knows he needs to get up, but he just can't. He rolls over and goes back to sleep, thinking that he will deal with all of this later, saying, "It is just too much."

The Practice

Here is how you address the difficulty of getting out of bed:

- **Be gentle and self-validate.** Talking to yourself harshly often makes you feel worse about yourself. Instead, gently look for the wisdom in your emotional experience. Ask yourself what emotions you are experiencing. Do they fit the situation in front of you? Would other people feel the same way if they were in similar circumstances? Give yourself permission to feel these feelings, and do so without judging them as good or bad. Stay away from judgments like telling yourself that you should feel differently or that your feelings are stupid.

- **Cheerlead.** Using encouraging statements can be a useful skill in motivating yourself to do something difficult (Linehan 1993a, 1993b). It is important to find phrases that motivate you but that do not sound inauthentic or forced. Some phrases to consider are "I can do this," or "This will be hard, but I feel better when I accomplish things during the day," or "I can take this day one moment at a time," or "Sometimes things turn out differently than I think they will." Consider crafting a few of your own cheerleading statements in times when you are not in distress, and practice them when your urges to avoid are high.

- **Identify the pros and cons of staying in bed.** It can be easy to identify many reasons why you should *not* get out of bed—but this reasoning will only keep you stuck. Open your mind to the benefits of getting out of bed and the downside of staying in bed. This helps you look at all sides of this decision. You may want to divide a piece of paper into two columns and write down your pros and cons. Next, evaluate each item on your list by asking yourself if it has a long or short impact on your life. Remember to generate as many pros and cons as you can. Stick to the facts and stay away from judgments.

- **Identify a reward.** Motivating yourself in the face of strong emotions is not easy. Sometimes it can be useful to identify what is in it for you to challenge yourself to get out of bed and face difficult situations. Ask yourself, "What is in it for me to get up and face the day?" If you cannot readily identify something, then create a reward for yourself. For example, say to yourself, "If I can get up and face this day, then at the end of the day I can take the evening off of homework, order dinner from my favorite restaurant, and then take a bath and relax." The challenge is to only give yourself the reinforcement if you complete the task. Each person's reward is unique, so be creative and find something that motivates you.

- **Connect with your long-term goals.** Staying in bed is probably not in line with your long-term goals, and in these moments that wisdom can be hard to remember. Ask yourself, "What are my long-term goals for work, school, and relationships?" Write these down. Remind yourself that these goals are important—despite your mood.

Checklist

☐   Have you validated your emotions?

☐   Are you encouraging yourself?

☐   Have you identified three benefits to getting out of bed?

☐   Have you set some personal rewards?

☐   Have you reminded yourself of your long-term goals?

32 · Prioritizing When Life Is Overwhelming

The Problem

It is easy for the tasks and demands of your life to feel overwhelming. Sometimes it may feel like you do not have time to get everything done, and you may feel lost, scared, and confused. You may not know where to start, or you may feel like your mind is spinning and you are paralyzed. When things feel overpowering, you may feel hopeless; you might want to give up and do nothing at all.

What It Looks Like

Christy is thirty-one years old and has worked hard to build a life for herself outside of treatment. She works twenty hours a week, takes a vocational class, and lives in an apartment with roommates. At times she struggles to balance her appointments, job, school, daily obligations, and relationships. When everything is in balance, Christy feels accomplished and independent. However, life can feel like too much when the scales are tipped.

It is Thursday evening, and Christy wants to give up. She has procrastinated all week on studying for an exam scheduled for Friday; her roommate's boyfriend has been living at their apartment in violation of an agreement, which is making her furious; she still needs to pay her phone bill before her phone gets shut off; and she is angry that her therapist canceled one of her sessions. If Christy does not get at least a C on the exam, she will fail her class; but everything else needs to get done as well. She has no idea where to start—it all feels like too much. She feels panic rising; resigned, she returns to the couch and turns on the TV. "I'm such a failure," she tells herself. "How did I ever think I could manage a normal life?"

The Practice

Here is how you address difficulties with prioritizing:

- **Notice and label your fear and anxiety.** Having difficulty knowing where to start can be scary and lead to avoidance or paralysis. Avoidance can happen very quickly, and before you know it you may have abandoned all of your tasks. Nonjudgmentally noticing and labeling your anxiety or fear will help you bring it into awareness; it will also help slow down the feelings. While it may seem counterintuitive, bringing your attention to an intense emotion in a nonjudgmental way (for example, saying to yourself, "I notice my heart beating quickly, I notice my palms sweating, I notice a fluttering feeling in my stomach") will begin the process of lowering the intensity. It will also help you identify which skills to try. This practice also stops the process of enhancing your anxiety, which is a natural consequence to judging it.

- **Identify your goals.** Identifying and remembering your goals helps ground you when you are having a difficult time prioritizing. Sometimes when you are overwhelmed you may notice thoughts like "I can't do this," "I don't know where to start," "It doesn't matter," "I don't care," or "I give up." Take a moment and turn your mind to your goals. Why is each of the tasks you have to do important? What is in it for you to complete them? Will you feel a sense of mastery? Will it move you closer to one of your long-term goals? Will it help support a relationship? It is important to focus on how battling through your fear will help you. Find a piece of paper or a journal and write down your goals.

- **Make a to-do list.** When you are overwhelmed, it can be tempting to start many tasks and give up before you have completed any one. You may find that just holding so many different things in your mind is creating more stress. Help yourself by getting out two sheets of paper. On the first page, write down all the tasks to be completed. Include both large and small tasks that are swirling around in your head. Next, indicate when each task must be completed. If there is no deadline, indicate the date you would like to complete it.

  Remember to distinguish what you *need* to complete from what you *want* to complete. Needs are the things you have to do in order to meet your responsibilities, like turning in a paper on time in order to get a grade. A want is something that is not absolutely necessary but something you'd simply like. Balancing needs and wants is a critical part of prioritizing (Linehan 1993a, 1993b). On the second piece of paper, rewrite your list in order of the date that tasks need to be completed. Now you have prioritized your tasks.

- **Breathe.** If you have a long list of things to do you, may notice your anxiety rising. Take a few minutes to do a breathing practice such as *ladder breathing* (inhale and say "one," exhale and say "one"; inhale and say "two," exhale and say "two"...all the way up to ten; when your mind wanders or you reach ten, begin again at one) or another mindful breathing practice that focuses your mind. If you practice mindful breathing while you look at your to-do list, you may notice your anxiety increase as you focus on the enormity of the task ahead of you, but if you continue to mindfully breathe, your anxiety will typically start decreasing and it will be easier to begin working. You can use this breathing practice when you notice your anxiety increasing as you tackle the list.

- **Practice one-mindfulness of your list.** *One-mindfulness* means doing just one thing in the moment. If you are eating, just eat. If you are reading, just read. If you are watching TV, just watch TV. Most of us tend to try to do too many things at once. Once you have prioritized your list, it is important to proceed one-mindfully, doing one task at a time (Linehan 1993a, 1993b). When you have completed a task, cross it off your list. Some people find that crossing things off their list gives them a sense of mastery and motivation to continue working. Notice when your mind wanders to a task farther down the list, and gently turn it back to the single task you are working on. Do your best to complete one task before moving on to the next. You are more efficient when you work one-mindfully.

Checklist

☐ Did you nonjudgmentally acknowledge your emotions?

☐ Have you identified your goals?

☐ Have you made your to-do list and placed the tasks in order by due date?

☐ Have you identified what you need to do versus what you want to do?

☐ Have you practiced mindful breathing?

CHAPTER 9

Drugs and Alcohol

33 · Drinking to Address Overwhelming Feelings

The Problem

You have found that alcohol is useful in controlling your emotions. While drinking may dull your sadness or loneliness, or make you feel more socially confident, once you sober up the feelings come back, sometimes with greater intensity. While you may feel that drinking helps you manage your emotions, using alcohol might make you even more vulnerable to extreme emotions, and this vulnerability can last for a few days after you have stopped drinking.

What It Looks Like

Mara is a twenty-seven-year-old who struggles with loneliness. She has worked hard to stay connected to a small group of friends. Mara is chronically anxious that she will do something to drive her friends away, as she has lost many friends in the past, sometimes from her behavior while drinking. As a result, she ends up feeling very anxious—sometimes so anxious that she cancels plans and stays home. Canceling her plans leaves her feeling deeply sad, lonely, and empty. Sometimes Mara's anxiety and loneliness feels unbearable. Mara enjoys drinking and feels that she has more fun when she can drink.

Tonight, Mara is getting ready to meet her friends, but she can't stop thinking about how everyone hates her and that she is too fat for all of her clothing. As her mind begins to spiral, she reaches for a glass of wine. She can feel her body relax soon after the first glass. Mara's friend arrives, and they continue to drink wine and chat. However, when Mara receives a text that her boyfriend will not be coming, she begins to get angry. She quickly fires off text message after text message demanding that he come, calling him names and threatening to break up with him. When he stops responding, Mara gets angrier and can't stop talking about how thoughtless her boyfriend is. "If he cared about me he would have come over," Mara yells, slurring her words. Now her friend is uncomfortable and wants to leave, which only enrages Mara more. As her friend leaves, Mara bursts into tears. Alone in her house, she now feels lonely and sad. She'll wake up hungover the next morning, feeling shame and regret.

The Practice

Here is how you manage feelings like anxiety, sadness, or loneliness without drinking:

- **Self-validate.** Ask yourself, "What is the wisdom in my experience? What about my feelings make sense? What are my emotions telling me that fit the situation?" Pay attention to your emotions; this is the first step in letting yourself experience them without reaching for alcohol to distract yourself or numb your experience.

- **Remind yourself that your emotions do not last forever.** Drinking alcohol will only put off experiencing these emotions. Ask yourself, "Do I want to feel like this later?" Consider the idea that the only way to the other side of a painful emotion is to go through that emotion and not avoid it.

- **Think about the consequences.** Think back to other times when you have used alcohol as a way to regulate your emotions. Ask yourself, "Were there any negative consequences?

Do I want to experience those consequences again?" Radically accept that alcohol may have more negative consequences for you than it does for other people in your life.

- **Stay connected.** Reach out to people in your life so that you feel connected. This can be hard when you are feeling anxious, sad, or lonely. Try initiating plans, and meet up with friends in places where you can do an activity other than drinking.

- **Try vigorous exercise.** Sometimes doing intense exercise can quickly shift your mood and help you ride out urges to use alcohol. Try running or doing jumping jacks, sit-ups, push-ups, or wall-sits. It is important to do something that gives you an intense sensation, which will help shift your emotional experience.

- **Contribute.** When you find yourself consumed by the intensity of your own experience, you can shift that by turning your focus toward someone else. Call someone you haven't spoken to in a while and ask him about his life, write a card to someone who is not well or someone you have lost touch with, visit an older relative, run an errand for someone, or write gratitude letters to those who have helped or supported you.

- **Remove alcohol from where you live.** Sometimes the most effective thing is to make alcohol more difficult to get. By removing it from your home you are creating a barrier between you and easily reaching for a drink. That is not to say that you couldn't go out and buy some or ask a friend to bring some over, but by adding a step to the process you are giving yourself more time to use skills first.

Checklist

☐ Have you self-validated?

☐ Have you removed alcohol from your house?

☐ Have you committed to trying something other than alcohol to change your mood, such as reaching out to a friend or exercising?

☐ Have you identified people in your life for whom you are grateful?

34 · USING RANDOM PILLS

The Problem

When emotions get overwhelming, you may look to anything to change the way that you feel. Sometimes that means taking random pills such as old prescriptions, over-the-counter medication for pain or sleep, or whatever is left in your medicine cabinet. You may take pills to take the edge off, to numb you out, or to make you fall asleep for an extended period of time. This decision can have negative consequences.

What It Looks Like

Patrick is a thirty-year-old who has struggled with regulating his emotions for much of his life. He takes prescribed medication daily, but sometimes he feels that it doesn't work. On this night, Patrick comes home from a difficult day at work and can't stop thinking about feedback from his boss on a report he had written. The conversation is on repeat in his mind. As the evening goes on, Patrick becomes more and more anxious that tomorrow, he'll be fired. He begins thinking about the other jobs that he lost, what an awful employee he is, and how no one will hire him. To him, life feels hopeless and terrifying. Patrick just wants the feelings to stop—he wants a break from life just for a little while. He goes into his bathroom and begins looking at what medications he has. His doctor has warned Patrick that his habit of taking over-the-counter sleeping, allergy, and pain medication is causing damage to his body. But at this moment he doesn't think about the consequences. "I just want to make this feeling go away and get to sleep," he tells himself before popping several pills.

The Practice

Here is how you can avoid taking random pills when feeling the urge to escape:

- **Identify your emotion.** Take a few minutes to be mindful of what you are feeling. Notice the sensations in your body. What urges do you have? Name the emotion or emotions that you are feeling.

- **Find compassion for yourself.** You must be feeling some very painful emotions. Be gentle, don't criticize or judge, slow down, and think about a way that you can self-soothe. Remind yourself that we all struggle. Ask yourself how you would help a friend in this situation, and then follow your advice.

- **Identify the long-term consequences.** Turn your mind toward the longer-term consequences of taking random pills. What have your doctors told you could happen as a result? Ask yourself, "Will taking pills solve the problem in the long term? Will the problem still be there tomorrow?"

- **Plan ahead.** Make a coping plan for future situations so that you have a strategy the next time you have urges to take random pills. Think about alternative skills to distract you or to decrease the intensity of painful emotions. Write them down, and keep your plan in a place that is easy to access when you are in distress. Consider sharing the plan with a friend who can help you when you are having a difficult time.

- **Be frank with your doctor.** Tell your doctor that using random pills is a behavior that you would like to work on. Ask her if there is a safe medication that you can take in situations when you feel like you need to decrease the intensity of your emotions quickly. Be open minded and curious during this conversation.

- **Remove pills from your home.** By removing pills from your home, you are creating a barrier that will prevent you from easily reaching for pills to regulate your emotions. This will help you slow down and take time to think about the pros and cons of using skills in the moment. Are you spending that extra time planning ways to get pills? Instead, use techniques described in this book to identify and regulate your emotions.

Checklist

☐ Have you identified the consequences?

☐ Have you removed random pills that you do not use from your house?

☐ Have you planned what skills to use in future situations?

35 · Using a Friend's Medication

The Problem

Sometimes taking a friend's medication can be tempting. Your friends may have prescription stimulants, benzodiazepines, or pain medications that seem like a good solution to your problem. While it can be dangerous to take medication that was not prescribed to you—perhaps because your own doctor doesn't recommend it for you—it can also stress, damage, and complicate the relationship with your friend.

What It Looks Like

Since she was young, Monique has had difficulty paying attention and completing tasks when she is anxious. She is easily distracted by her emotions, which come in intense waves. Monique is a diligent seventeen-year-old student who wants to do well, but her emotions make her life and performance in school unpredictable and inconsistent. Monique has had a difficult week fighting with her boyfriend and feeling left out by her friends. She has a big paper to complete and wants to get some stimulants from a friend to help her complete her work. She also likes that stimulants decrease her appetite. Monique has called her friend many times in the past asking for the medication; they used to spend a lot of time together, but during the past few months they have seen less of each other. Monique asked her doctor if he would prescribe the stimulant, but he said no, suspecting that the medication ultimately makes her anxiety worse.

Monique calls her friend and leaves a message but doesn't hear back that day. She calls again the next day, and her friend picks up and sounds irritated. She agrees to give Monique a few pills but asks that she not call her again. Monique apologizes but feels that she really needs the medication. Monique is grateful to have the pills but soon feels anxious that she has lost another relationship and done something that goes against her values.

The Practice

Here is how you can manage the stressors of life without taking a friend's pills:

- **Attend to vulnerability factors.** Rather than relying on other people's drugs, take care of yourself. Pay attention to what makes you emotionally vulnerable—and address those factors. When in balance, the following elements will help you be in better emotional control: Getting enough sleep—typically eight to ten hours is what most people need—eating balanced meals, exercising, taking only necessary medications, and attending to any physical illness you may have. Also, it is important to not take alcohol, weed, cocaine, or other drugs, especially if these drugs cause severe mood swings.

- **Prioritize.** Think about your priorities. What is more important to you in the long run: getting pills or the relationship you have with your friend? Remember to consider the long-term versus short-term benefits of your behavior.

- **Review your values.** Ask yourself, "Does this behavior go against my values?" Taking medication from other people means that they will have less than they are prescribed. It also means that you are asking them to be dishonest with their own doctors. It means that both of you must keep a secret. Crossing your values repeatedly can create a cycle of shame and guilt that can be depleting and lead to increased self-loathing and self-hatred.

- **Find an alternative solution to your problem.** Spend some time thinking about alternatives that could help you regulate your emotions and attention. Can you build more structure around the task you must complete or the emotion you want to regulate more effectively? Do you need to do more planning or take more time? Can you meet with a doctor to get more information about ways to manage your emotions or attention? Could you work with a provider to get your own prescription? Consider alternatives that do not damage your relationships or cause you to feel shame or guilt.

Checklist

☐ Have you asked yourself what impact taking your friend's medication will have on your friendship?

☐ Have you clarified your values around asking for someone else's medication?

☐ Have you identified vulnerability factors that you could work on?

CHAPTER 10

Urges to Lash Out

The Problem

You are extremely angry at someone close to you. You are so upset that you are on the verge of physically attacking him. You know that it is not the right thing to do, but you feel that he deserves it for whatever it is he has done.

It is important to recognize that anger is a common human experience. We all experience it. Ultimately becoming abusive or violent is a choice rather than an inevitability, however.

What It Looks Like

Jonas, a twenty-five-year-old construction worker with BPD, woke up in a bad mood. He had not slept well after a fight with his girlfriend, and he was not looking forward to work. Yesterday, the general contractor on a big home-renovation project blamed Jonas for having done shoddy work on a deck; he wanted him to redo a section Jonas had spent hours on the previous day. As Jonas drove up to the construction site, he saw his boss laughing it up with some of the other workers. His blood began to boil. He thought to himself, "If my boss chews me out today, I am going to slap him silly."

The Practice

Before you do anything else, make sure that you are not in a situation where you can directly attack the person. If the person is not in your presence, then follow the steps below. If the person is in your presence, then leave immediately. If you cannot leave, place all your focus on your breath and do so until you can leave.

1. **Acknowledge and validate your feelings.** The healthy first step is simply to acknowledge and validate that you feel hurt and angry. This is not as simple as it sounds, because when you get angry, acknowledging that you feel hurt by another person can make you feel vulnerable and exposed—it may be that all you can think about in the moment is your desire for revenge and to do something that shows that you won't take things lying down. The problem is that revenge perpetuates anger because it never allows you to examine how you got to anger in the first place.

2. **Acknowledge your vulnerability factors.** Once you have validated your feelings, notice your vulnerability factors such as being tired, feeling hurt or upset by unrelated matters, feeling angry about situations that included the other person, or feeling other emotions. Again, this is acknowledging that it makes sense that you feel the way that you do.

3. **Use calming techniques.** Slow deep breathing, in particular, is an effective and easy calming technique. Take in a deep breath and hold it, then breathe out slowly through pursed lips and pause. Do this until the intensity of the tension diminishes. Other options to calm yourself down are to notice the tension in your shoulders and arms and then relax those muscles. Also, you cannot be extremely cold and angry at the same time. Imagine being very angry and then jumping into an ice-cold shower or lake. Your body goes into self-preservation mode, and the emotion of anger takes a backseat to dealing with the cold. If it is a cold day, take off your sweater or coat and stand outside. If it is a warm day, consider taking a cold shower.

4. **Forgive.** Forgiveness is very difficult whether you have BPD or not; it's also, ultimately, the most powerful thing you can do. To forgive someone means making a conscious decision to not only set aside any plans of revenge for the hurt the other person did to you, but to move on with compassion and wish that the other person recognizes his hurtful behavior and apologizes for what he has done. Importantly, you cannot forgive someone until you fully recognize the hurt the other person has caused and the hurt that you feel. Holding on to resentment has serious psychological and physical consequences for your health. Practicing forgiveness not only helps heal the relationship, it also helps heal your mind and body.

Keep in mind that another thing that does not work is taking out your anger on something else, like a pillow. In fact, expressing your anger against inanimate objects won't make you less angry at all. Research shows that hitting a punching bag or sofa cushion actually increases rather than diminishes anger (Bushman 2002). It doesn't work because you are training your brain to associate anger with aggression rather than with reconciliation and kindness.

Checklist

☐ Have you acknowledged that you are angry?

☐ Have you identified your vulnerability factors?

☐ Have you used calming techniques?

☐ Have you forgiven the other person?

37 · The Urge to Punch a Wall

The Problem

You are beyond angry at something that you feel is unfair. You are overwhelmed by the urge to punch the wall in front of you. You have done this in the past, and, while it felt good in the moment, it has led to visits to the emergency room and many holes in the wall. Sometimes you experience the feeling of trying to hold the anger in, only to explode hours later. You may have been told that you have an anger problem—and even though this may be true, someone telling you that can make you even angrier.

What It Looks Like

Jim, an eighteen-year-old with BPD, was referred to us by his primary care clinician after a third incident of having to cast his right hand. He had broken his hand on two occasions and had had multiple X-rays for suspected breaks after punching walls. Jim admits that he has a very difficult time controlling his anger and that at times he wants to punch anything, even people; however, he knows that he doesn't want to hurt anyone else and that punching walls "gets the anger out." Mostly the anger comes out when someone pisses him off or when he feels shame that he has done something wrong.

The Practice

If you can step back and look at the behavior of punching walls, often it seems disproportionate to the situation—even if at the time it felt just right. Use the mnemonic **LET GO** to avoid the urge to hit a wall:

- Leave. When you notice an urge to punch a wall—or anything else for that matter—go to a place where there isn't a wall, or where it would be very socially inappropriate to punch a wall. For instance, walk outside where there are no walls, or go to your local coffee shop, where social expectations would stop you from punching any walls in public.

- Express. Now that you are in a place where you are less likely to punch something, express your feelings to yourself. When you are in a calmer state, let the other person know that you are angry. Be clear as to the situation that made you angry.

- Take an ice-cold shower. It is virtually impossible to be angry and freezing. This is a tried-and-tested intervention—even our angriest of patients have told us that they are far less angry after getting out of a freezing shower.

- Get active. Use intense exercise to burn off angry energy. Go for a hard run. Do as many sit-ups as you can. Skip—you can't be angry and skip.

- Openness to fun. Humor is an excellent intervention when you are angry. Watch a funny movie, sitcom, or online video.

Checklist

☐ Have you identified that you are angry?

☐ Have you used LET GO?

38 · THE URGE TO DESTROY ANOTHER PERSON'S PROPERTY

The Problem

You are angry at someone and want to get revenge. You know that she has a special connection to some item important to her: a brand-new TV, her mother's china collection, a favorite piece of jewelry. All you want to do is destroy that special thing to get back at her.

What It Looks Like

Forty-two-year-old Henrietta, who has BPD, has been married to her husband for four years. She is extremely jealous of his relationship with his parents, because she perceives that they don't like her and that they have never accepted her as his wife. Her in-laws are visiting the couple and have offered to take them out for dinner. Henrietta is getting agitated. She does not like that her husband feels as close to his parents as he does, feeling that any love that he has for them takes away from the love he has for her. Her husband puts on a tie that his father bought him for his birthday some years ago, and her anger is so strong that she wants to cut the tie in half and smash the framed photograph of her in-laws that sits on the couple's piano. She wants to smash the piano as well. Henrietta knows that these actions will hurt her husband, but she feels that at least then he would understand just how much she does not like his parents and that perhaps he would have less of a desire to spend any time with them.

The Practice

The intense desire to harm someone else's property can be avoided with these practices:

- **Acknowledge your anger.** As with the other anger scenarios, knowing that you are angry and noticing the urge to destroy property is the first step in dealing with potential harmful behavior.

- **Recognize your bodily reactions.** Most people with a history of acting on their urges to destroy things have a habitual and physical pattern of anger. What's your typical reaction? Your body sensations are often the first clue. You might, for instance, have noticed a flare of rage rushing through your body, your heart beating faster, your jaw clenching. The sooner you can tell that you are getting angry, the more time you have to prevent acting on your urges.

- **Restrain your hands.** If you are about to smash a TV, vase, telephone, or some other object, hold one hand down with your other one. Clench your fist so that you cannot pick up the object. Sit on your hands, or lie on the ground and commit to not getting up until the urge diminishes.

- **Sit down and breathe.** It doesn't matter if you are in your kitchen, at work, or at a social event—just sit down and breathe. This action gives you the time to turn the anger down, and you can't break things if you're sitting away from them.

- **Leave the crowd.** If you're around other people, walk out of the space you are in. Again, this action buys you the time that you need to lower your level of anger and consider alternative ways to express of your feelings.

Checklist

- ☐ Have you identified that you are angry by noticing your emotions and urges?

- ☐ Are you restraining yourself?

- ☐ Are you buying yourself the time necessary to consider alternatives?

39 · THE URGE TO INSULT OR DEVALUE ANOTHER

The Problem

You are very angry at someone, and you have a strong urge to insult or devalue her in a way that you know will really sting. Perhaps you want to say something denigrating about a particular weakness or vulnerability that she has. You may want her to feel just as bad as you do. You might want to say things like, "You are the worst parent ever," or "You are a terrible therapist" or "You are a lousy lover— anybody would be better than you." You might even get away with your actions if the person you're speaking to is of trivial importance in your life; but lashing out or devaluing a person can be relationship-destroying if the targeted person is important to you.

What It Looks Like

Thirty-two-year-old Nancy broke up with her girlfriend several weeks ago. They had agreed to stay friends, and so far their relationship has been good. But then Nancy's ex went to Miami on vacation and posted pictures of her trip on Facebook. She clearly appeared to be having fun. Nancy feels left out; she also feels hurt that her ex never had fun with her. Now she wants to call her ex and tell her how fat she looks in the pictures, knowing just how badly she feels about her weight and that she would suffer hearing her mention it.

The Practice

Often the urge to lash out and insult or devalue is fueled by anger or feeling hurt. At times, this can trigger the desire to get even or take revenge on the person who hurt you. To avoid the intense urge to insult or devalue someone, practice these techniques:

- **Validate yourself.** As with many of the techniques in this book, the first step to avoiding the urge to lash out at someone is self-validation. It makes perfect sense that you would feel hurt if you had either been verbally attacked yourself or if you imagined that the other person was doing something to hurt you on purpose. The desire to lash out is understandable.

- **Understand the facts.** Once you have self-validated, ask yourself the following questions:

  What is the emotion I am feeling?

  How did it arise?

  What do I feel like doing or saying to the other person?

  What is my goal in the relationship?

  Is what I am about to say in keeping with that goal?

- **Take a balanced view.** What is each person's perspective? In some circumstances we have been told that not lashing out means that the other person "wins." The truth is that when you lash out, everyone loses. The other person is hurt and does not like being with you; and often what you say crosses your values, and you end up feeling shame. On the other hand, you don't want the other person to get away with what she did or what you imagined she did. Insulting or demeaning someone is not skillful. It's also ineffective in the long term—and if you decide to do so, there will be negative consequences.

- **Talk it out.** Once you have taken the steps to figure out how you got to this point, then you can act—and hopefully with self-respect. Once you are less angry, explain to the person how what she did or said resulted in the way that you are feeling. Then let the person know that the relationship is important to you and that you do not want to make the situation worse.

- **Troubleshoot for a future situation.** If it is likely that such circumstances will arise again, plan how you'll cope and what you might do differently next time. If the person loves you and is interested in your healing from BPD, she will appreciate the effort you are making and recognize that you are doing something different, something other than devaluing or insulting her.

Checklist

☐ Have you identified the emotion you are feeling right now?

☐ Did you consider the factors that got you to this point?

☐ Have you stated your goal in the relationship?

☐ Have you talked to the other person?

☐ Have you devised a plan for ways to cope in the future?

CHAPTER 11

Negative Self-Thoughts

The Problem

You hate yourself. You hate everything about who you are. You hate how you think. You hate what you do to others in relationships. You hate your very essence.

What It Looks Like

Twenty-seven-year-old Shayna, a receptionist at a health club, says, "I just think about how much I hate everything: my body, my disorder, my attitude, my decisions, my life, how I destroy relationships. Even when I feel better and less hateful, I'm still not happy with who I am… It's hard to explain. At times I feel like I deserve nothing, and at other times I don't feel like I am a person at all, like someone so worthless cannot be real."

The negative thought of self-loathing is one of the more unrelenting and destructive thoughts in BPD.

The Practice

Here is how you address feelings of self-hatred:

- **Have patience.** You have likely spent many years in self-loathing. Creating new brain pathways and new ways of thinking takes time and practice. This is the way the brain works! Being patient as you use the following skills is the first act of loving yourself.

- **Ask for help.** Seek assistance not only from your friends and family but from teachers, therapists, priests, religious leaders, coworkers, and self-help groups. Focusing on getting help for yourself is an act of kindness to yourself, and if you have professional help the specific work is just about you.

- **Don't avoid the self-loathing.** Unless you face the pain that self-loathing brings, you cannot address it. Somewhere in your life you went from being a child who had no concept of self-hatred to hating yourself. You weren't born this way. Facing this fact is painful, and yet it is the only way to get out of it. Do this by simply acknowledging that the pain is there—don't dwell on it or ruminate. In fact, when you can face the pain without dwelling on it, you are mastering it and healing from the self-hatred.

- **Forgive and forgive and forgive.** You must forgive yourself for all your misdeeds and perceived misdeeds. If you have crossed your values and hurt someone, then ask him for forgiveness as well. At any point in time you are doing the best you can do. You will do better as you become more skillful. Forgiveness of yourself is a practice in self-compassion.

- **Be with people you love and do things you enjoy.** Do you like reading? Read. Do you enjoy playing a musical instrument? Play on. Do you love dancing? Join a dance class. Do you take pleasure in being with a certain group of friends? Set up a weekly dinner. The more you practice doing things you love, the more you will love; this is the opposite of punishing yourself because of self-loathing, which deprives you of the things you love.

- **Try a Zen practice.** Another way to tackle the problem of self-hatred is through this common Zen skill: Think about someone you respect whom you consider to be a wise, compassionate person. Now, imagine that person living with you in your mind and body during moments of self-loathing, and

153

see how he might handle your self-hatred. This is a difficult task, but with practice you will find greater self-compassion.

Checklist

☐ Are you being patient?

☐ Are you forgiving yourself?

☐ Are you doing the things you love?

41 · COMPARING YOURSELF TO OTHERS

The Problem

You find that you are always comparing yourself to other people in your life. You have been doing it for years. In each comparison you find yourself not as smart, not as pretty, not as creative, not as interesting, not as special, not as good a friend, and so on and so on.

These types of comparisons can lead to dangerous spirals in thinking that drive self-loathing, self-hatred, hopelessness, and dangerous and self-destructive behavior.

What It Looks Like

Twenty-nine-year-old Leela, who runs her own catering company, received a lunch invitation from a friend who wanted Leela to meet a few of her coworkers. Leela was anxious about the lunch plan and thought a lot about what she would wear and what she would talk about. She also noticed worry thoughts about being judged by these new people, but she was eager to make some new friends.

Leela arrives at the lunch date and immediately has a difficult time paying attention. Her mind is racing as she looks at how pretty and smart the other women are. "Why would these women like someone like me?" Leela says to herself. "I have nothing important to say… I am such a fraud." Leela's friend asks her why she is so quiet. Leela just smiles and tries to enter into the conversation. But her mind goes blank as she looks around the table. "There is no way they will like me. They are clearly more successful and have more friends." Leela can't slow down her thoughts. As the meal ends, she realizes that she doesn't feel like she connected with anyone. "What is wrong with me?" she begins to wonder. "I really am horrible! Of course no one wants to talk to me. If I were interesting they would have engaged me in conversation. Perhaps if I were smarter and prettier they would have liked me better. People like me don't deserve to have these opportunities, as all I do is focus on myself anyway. How can I ever keep up with women like them: beautiful, smart, and fun? Someone like me never stood a chance."

The Practice

Here is how you address the issue of constantly comparing yourself to others.

- **Notice comparison thoughts.** The first step in battling comparison thoughts is to be aware that you are engaging in comparing behavior. This may sound easy; however, if you have developed a habit for this type of thinking you may engage in comparison thinking almost automatically. Think about the type of comparisons that you make. Do you tend to compare yourself to others based on appearance? Intelligence? Skill level? In which situations are you at highest risk for comparing yourself? Consider in what environments you find yourself using comparisons the most. Once you identify common comparison thoughts, these will be your red flags for comparison thinking. When you notice the thoughts, say to yourself, "Comparison thought." This will slow down the chain of thinking and help your mind not get more caught up in the content of your thinking. Once you have labeled the thought, turn your mind back to the conversation or what you are working on. You will need to practice doing this over and over again.

- **Identify your emotions and validate yourself.** Comparison thoughts are typically tied closely to strong emotions. Comparisons can create a powerful distraction from your emotions. Consider what emotions drive your comparison thoughts. Think about how your mind reacts to fear, sadness, shame, jealousy, and envy. Once you have identified the emotions, use validation to remind yourself about the wisdom in your experience. For example, it makes sense that Leela would feel anxious and doubt herself when meeting new people, especially when she is really hoping to create new relationships. Sometimes, validating the emotion (not the comparison thoughts!) will slow you down and help you focus on your feelings instead of getting caught up in destructive thinking.

- **Shift your attention by turning your mind.** After you have noticed that you are engaging in comparisons, and after you have validated your emotions, you must commit to shifting your attention. In DBT, this skill is called Turning the Mind (Linehan 1993a, 1993b). The challenge with this practice is that comparisons can have a powerful grip on your attention. Identify a place to turn your mind. For Leela, it was shifting her attention back to the conversation. When your mind wanders to comparisons, notice it, then gently turn it back to the topic at hand. It can be helpful to fully engage as soon as you turn your attention back. For example, Leela could turn her attention back to the lunch conversation and immediately ask someone a question or make a statement; this is a quick way for her to become an active participant instead of just an observer. This will help focus your mind on the present.

- **Balance the comparison and find the other side.** If you compare yourself to others often, it's likely that your practice is one-sided. That is, you are very skilled at finding yourself on the negative side of the comparison. Try something new: Practice balancing your comparisons. For every negative comparison, challenge yourself to find the other side.

- **Compare yourself to an earlier you.** One of the most challenging DBT skills—and one that's very effective—is the comparison skill in the Distress Tolerance Module of the DBT protocol (Linehan 1993a, 1993b). This skill asks you to compare your present self with your past self during a time when you were struggling. This skill takes practice, but once mastered it can be very successful at lowering your distress. For example, you could look back and say, "One year ago, when I was in distress, I did not know skills. Now when I face this challenge I may still struggle, but I am doing so skillfully instead of using destructive behaviors."

Checklist

☐ Have you identified comparison thoughts?

☐ Have you self-validated?

☐ Have you taken the other side of the comparison?

42 · FEELING LIKE NOBODY LOVES YOU OR CARES ABOUT YOU

The Problem

You feel that nobody loves you and that no one will ever care about you. You might also feel that if people *really* knew you, they couldn't possibly love you. You might have feelings of aloneness, hopelessness, and despair—and this can be an unbearable experience.

What It Looks Like

Atticus is a forty-year-old man with BPD who feels unloved. He doesn't believe it when people tell him that they love him. He suspects that they only say so because they "have to." He says that his parents tell him they care "because they are my parents," and his boyfriend says so "because he wants to reassure me," and his therapist tells him that "because she tells all her clients that."

The Practice

Here are some ways to change your thinking that no one loves or cares about you:

- **Notice your negative thoughts.** Feeling unloved is actually a thought and not a feeling. The feeling you have might be anger or sadness. The statement "No one loves me"—unless you have actual data that no one loves you—is the conclusion that you come to when you experience disconnection from the people who you love. A more accurate statement would be: "I am noticing the thought that I hate myself. I notice thinking that people don't really love me, even when they tell me they do. I notice skepticism when they tell me they do, and so I have come to the conclusion that I am unlovable and that no one will ever care about me." This is a bit of a mouthful to say; however, slowing down and seeing just how you came to the conclusion that no one loves you will give you important information about how you think and the habitual nature of destructive thoughts. The bottom line is that feeling unloved is something that happens inside your head.

- **Practice and have patience.** Because the idea that you are unlovable has taken years to develop, it will take some time to undo. When you have the automatic and habitual thought that you are unlovable and that no one will ever care about you, *stop!* Tell yourself that this is only a thought, not a matter of fact. You have to believe that you are loved even when it doesn't feel that way. Say to yourself: "I am loved, even though I don't feel loved."

- **Be kind.** Think about how wonderful it feels when people do nice things for you. When you practice acts of love, compassion, and kindness, people cannot help but love you! You don't have to be kind to everyone, particularly if they have hurt you. Find someone you know who deserves your love and compassion. Be kind to someone in need. Call a friend and tell her you care about her.

- **Forgive.** If you feel unloved because you feel hurt or rejected by the behavior of someone you are close to, learn to forgive her and also to forgive yourself. Forgiveness is a powerful way to change the intensity of an overwhelming feeling.

Checklist

- [ ] Have you labeled your unlovable feeling as a thought and not as a fact?

- [ ] Have you told yourself that you know you are loved and that you are surrounded by love?

- [ ] Have you practiced an act of kindness and compassion today?

- [ ] Have you forgiven the other person and yourself?

43 · Feeling Toxic

The Problem

You feel that you are a toxic person and that every relationship you have turns bad because you are in it. When you think about yourself in a relationship, you feel that you have nothing to give. You define yourself as an unsupportive, draining, unrewarding, clingy, unsatisfying, demanding, and demeaning person. Because of this, you don't want people in your life; you imagine that you'll end up poisoning them.

What It Looks Like

When Janet turned thirty-five, she finally opened up to the idea that she could date someone. Prior to that, she considered herself to be too toxic to be of much worth to anyone. As she started to date, she noticed old feelings begin to creep in. Janet would go on a few dates, and the minute she noticed clinginess, neediness, or being a "parasite," she would call it off and try again with another person. She began to imagine herself as a poison in the relationship. Janet figures that she'll end up destroying anyone she dates. She gives evidence that she is toxic: One man she dated lost his job. Another had a skiing accident. A third was arrested for drinking and driving. Janet imagines that these facts are all proof of her toxicity, and she discounts any positives that happened in the lives of others as luck.

The Practice

Feeling toxic is typically triggered by something interpersonal. As with many practices in this book, you must pay attention to the experience you are having in order to deal with it. Here are the necessary steps to overcome feeling like you might be toxic:

- **Identify the triggers.** Take a moment to step back and breathe. Think in detail about the incident that triggered the thought that you are toxic. Describe what actually happened as accurately as you can. Use facts of the scenario; avoid making judgments.

- **Locate the emotion physically.** Notice the physical experiences in your body. Are your muscles tense? Are your fists clenched? Be as precise as you can be. Put words to the physical effects on your body. Also describe any self-judgments you are having.

- **Own the experience.** The painful feelings you experience are *your* feelings. These feelings are happening inside your mind and body in the present moment, even if in the present moment you are simply sitting and watching TV. The experience of toxicity is internal to you, and unless you share it with someone it's not something that an outsider can see.

- **Tell another story.** You have a choice in how you interpret situations and in how you respond to your sense of self as toxic. By owning your feelings, you gain the power to change them and then reduce the amount of suffering you experience. Rather than tell yourself that you are toxic, realize that you are a tiny fraction of the entire universe and that you don't have the power to destroy lives. Realize that you are not responsible for others' choices and that they can make decisions for themselves.

- **Release the toxicity.** Focus your attention on the toxic thought and breathe with awareness. With every exhalation, have an intention of releasing the toxicity. For the next few minutes, feel the toxicity leaving your body with every exhalation. If it helps, imagine that you are breathing your toxicity into the consuming power of the sun.

Checklist

☐ Have you pinpointed the triggers?

☐ Have you accurately described the triggering experience?

☐ Did you localize the feeling in your body and mind?

☐ Have you breathed out your toxicity?

CHAPTER 12

Living in the Past or in the Future

The Problem

Many people with BPD cannot imagine a future without enduring suffering. Some teenagers with BPD, for example, cannot imagine living beyond their twentieth birthday. Living in fear of the future often leads to being stuck and not doing the things necessary to move on. And this is often made worse when the friends in your life are moving on and you aren't. If you are perfectionistic, the fear of failure compounds the fear of the future; rather than trying and failing, you don't try at all. The fear of what may happen in the coming years starts to creep in and there seems to be no escape.

What It Looks Like

Bobby is twenty-two and has just completed his sophomore year in college. A series of withdrawals and medical leaves of absence has slowed his progress through the academic phase of his life. As he starts his junior year, he thinks about what he will do after college. Thinking about his future sickens him, and Bobby notices the urge to not go to class or get any of his assignments in. He begins to have a series of catastrophizing thoughts about a two-page essay due in two weeks: "I'm certain that I won't get an A…so I won't do the assignment…which means I'll fail the class…which means that I won't graduate…and therefore I won't get a job…and therefore I won't have money for an apartment…and I'll be living in a homeless shelter or on the streets for the rest of my life."

The Practice

Typically, the reason for your fear of the future is that you are looking at it through the lens of the struggles of the past and the experience of an anxiety-filled present. Here is how to move away from your intense fear of the future:

- **Understand that the future is not real.** In order to start addressing this fear, you have to recognize that, by definition, the future is never real and it never comes. It is a concept of the mind, and your mind can create infinite futures, even wonderful ones. At the core of your fear of the future—which your mind has fabricated—is the belief that, if a certain outcome happens, you will not be able to cope with it. Even if what you think is not real, your imagination is very real and has very real effects. Unless you pay attention and deal with your fear of the future, you run the risk of creating self-fulfilling prophecies. It makes perfect sense that you would have anxiety about what your future holds, but dealing with what *is* rather than with what you fear (what *is not*) gives you the best chance of getting out of suffering.

- **Identify the fear.** What is it about the present moment that makes you fear the future? Define it. Describe it. Bobby has gone from having a required assignment due in two weeks to living in a homeless shelter. If somehow that were true, it would make sense to fear the future, but all he knows in the present moment is that he has an assignment due. All the rest his mind has created. To identify his fear, Bobby might say simply, "I fear not getting an A."

- **Identify the warning.** Fear is the body's way of warning you about something. For instance, fearing a poisonous snake is your body and brain's way of warning you against getting too close—because if you are bitten you may get very sick or possibly die, and so fear of the snake makes sense. In Bobby's case he might say, "The fear of not getting an A is warning me that I risk failing the class and lowering my GPA. It's a warning to start studying and writing early."

- **Identify your action urge.** What is your mind and body telling you to do? In Bobby's case he might say, "Because I fear not getting an A on my paper, and therefore have the fear of my peers and family seeing me as a failure, I don't even want to start writing. My urge is to stay in my room and not write."

- **Identify the consequence of following your action urge.** Is the consequence of your automatic response consistent with your long-term goals? In Bobby's case, he wants to graduate from college. Staying in his room and not completing his paper is not consistent with his goal of earning a degree. Completing the paper and risking getting a B or a C will probably mean that he still passes the class and stays on the path to graduation. Not completing the paper is more likely to lead to his failing and therefore not graduating.

- **Act as if you are not afraid.** Once you have gone through the above steps, act opposite to your urge. If you fear you won't get a promotion at work, and your automatic urge is to not try as hard or skip work altogether, your opposite action would be to get to work on time every day and try even harder! In Bobby's case, he would leave his room, perhaps ask a friend to go to the library with him, and start writing a few sentences. Each time the fear sets in, Bobby would again use the skill of opposite action to write a few more sentences, keeping his long-term goals in mind.

Checklist

☐ Have you identified the fear and its warning?

☐ Have you identified your action urge?

☐ Have you thought about what the consequences will be if you act on your urge?

☐ Are you acting opposite to the urge?

45 · Fear of Never Getting Better

The Problem

You have had a particularly rough week. Suddenly it seems that all the gains you have made have evaporated. You feel that you are back at square one and that you will never get better.

What It Looks Like

Jeremy, a thirty-eight-year-old with BPD, has had years of different therapies and medications that he feels have not been useful. When he started DBT, he finally felt that he found a therapy that worked. He even believes that DBT has changed his life. During the last week, though, he broke up with his girlfriend and now feels angry and sad, and wants to start drinking again. He now comes into therapy saying that he will never get better. "What's the point in even trying?" Jeremy laments. "Therapy is never going to work. I'm never going to get better."

The Practice

It makes perfect sense that you would have anxiety about what your future holds, that you wonder if your pain will ever go away and whether your treatment will be effective. But when this fear consumes the present moment and hinders progress, it's time to get help. Learning to tolerate your fear that you will not get better is a multi-step process:

- **Understand that the future is unknown.** Future-focused fears can be very painful. But the reality is that everyone must live with and practice acceptance around the idea that the future is unknown. Getting used to the idea that the future is uncertain can feel intolerable. Yet, when your mind begins to live in a dreaded future, you suffer a future that has not yet happened—and you run the risk of creating painful self-fulfilling prophecies. If you become too frightened and anxious about getting better, you will not be able to be in the present—or use your therapy, or practice your skills. It is helpful to remember that the only time you need to be in the future is to plan a goal; and worrying is not planning.

- **Validate your fear.** Whether they have BPD or not, many people fear the future. An important step is to confirm that your fear makes sense. This is where you use your self-validation skills to remind yourself that there is wisdom in your fear. For instance, if no therapy has ever worked for you before, it makes sense that you would fear that the current therapy won't work for you either. Remember: Seeing the wisdom in your emotion does not mean allowing your emotion to take over. It simply means acknowledging that the emotion is there.

- **Assess the present, not the future.** Once you have validated your fear, you must bring yourself back to the present moment and nonjudgmentally see how your fear of the future fits with your current experience. Check the facts of your situation by asking yourself, "What am I doing now in the present to help myself get better?" If you are not in therapy, ask yourself, "Given how I am struggling, are there behaviors that are keeping me stuck in suffering? Am I repeating past behaviors that I know have not helped me but can't stop myself from doing because of habit or because I don't know what else to do?" Keep a daily diary of such behaviors to track them. After a while you will begin to notice a pattern.

- **Use more DBT skills.** If you are in DBT, are you sticking to your commitment to get better by attending therapy, completing your diary card, taking your medication, exercising, and taking time to do the things you enjoy? If you are slipping in your commitment, then take this opportunity to try one skill on your own or review and complete your diary card. Think about a time in the last week when you have used skills or done something differently and felt effective. As your anxiety decreases in the moment, try one of your skills for tolerating distress to distract yourself a bit. Remember to go back to self-validation and checking the facts when this worry returns.

- **Avoid catastrophizing.** Fear that you will never get better is a fear that will likely come and go throughout the treatment process, particularly when you are in difficult situations or when you are experiencing intense emotions. Fear of the future is a practice—albeit an ineffective one—so the more you practice effectively staying present with this fear and not catastrophizing, the more skilled and effective you will get at managing it.

Checklist

☐   Have you validated your fears?

☐   Are you staying present?

☐   Are you noticing and avoiding catastrophizing?

46 · Continuing to Replay the Past

The Problem

You hold on to and relive negative experiences or memories of the past, memories associated with emotions that hurt you. You keep replaying arguments or discussions that left a painful emotional imprint in your mind, and the reliving keeps you stuck in the past. (This problem is separate from trauma and PTSD, which require dedicated treatment.)

What It Looks Like

Kathleen is a very sensitive seventeen-year-old with BPD who is working on being able to experience and tolerate her emotions without becoming self-destructive. During therapy, she is always engaged and chatty, but whenever her mother comes to a session, Kathleen refuses to talk. In individual sessions, Kathleen expresses deep love for her mother, so her behavior when her mother is in the room is confusing. Her mother says that she and Kathleen had been extremely close until Kathleen had turned fourteen. That was when Kathleen's mother had lost her own mother to cancer. She notes that Kathleen had also been close to her grandmother but has appeared to have dealt with her grandmother's death as well as could be expected.

"When my grandmother died," Kathleen finally admits, "I went to my mother and gave her a hug. My mother was crying and was so sad. As she was crying, she talked about her mother and about how empty she felt, that she had lost everything and that now she had no one." Kathleen says that when she heard her mother say that she had no one, she felt more hurt than ever before. "How could my mother feel that she has no one? She has me. How could she possibly say something like that?"

Whenever Kathleen sees her mother cry, it triggers the memory of her mother saying that she has no one. That memory is tied to powerful and intolerable feelings of loneliness and sadness, which have led Kathleen to engage in self-destructive behaviors as a way to manage her pain. She has never told her mother about her feelings and the reasons for them; she's held on to the memory and associated emotions for more than three years.

The Practice

The only way to get out of the past is to move to the present. Simple as that! However, that straightforward wisdom can be difficult to practice without help from some of these techniques:

- **Accept the past.** Acceptance is the first step to letting go of a painful past. For Kathleen, wishing that her mother had never said what she said will not change what happened. Accept that everything you once had and everything you have now all led to who you are today—the good *and* the bad.

- **Distance yourself from the pain.** Doing so will bring clarity. Take a break and explore something else for a while; doing so will yield new experiences, which will lead to your seeing the past through a different perspective. Going back to a painful memory is very different from never having left it in the first place.

- **Focus on what can change.** What Kathleen's mother said will never change. What has happened in your past won't either. Focus exclusively on what you *can* change. If you can't change a past experience, then change the way you think about it.

- **Know that you are responsible for you.** You are in full control of your life, your thoughts, and your reactions to experiences. No one can force you to see things in a certain way. You may want to blame the rest of the world, but giving others responsibility for your experience disempowers you. Kathleen is responsible for changing how she reacts to her mother's words.

- **Recognize that today is not the time of the past event.** For Kathleen to deny that things are different in this present moment than they were years ago would not be useful. Such denial would keep her trapped. She is older and wiser. Speaking to her mother about her past hurt would bring the Kathleen that she is today into the present moment, a moment she can actually deal with.

- **Focus on this present moment.** You are totally capable of making the decision right now that the painful experiences from your past will not predict your future. What are you going to do differently from what you have done in the past? Rather than shying away from her mother, Kathleen should realize that it's time to have a discussion with her. In fact, when Kathleen eventually talked to her mother, her mother broke down and cried, "You suffered for so long! Why didn't you ever tell me? Of course, I didn't mean that I was alone from you. I'm so sad that you thought that."

Checklist

☐ Have you accepted that what happened in the past has happened?

☐ Are you focusing on what you can change?

☐ Are you bringing your attention to the present moment and what you can do differently?

CHAPTER 13

Paranoia

47 · Feeling Like People Are Doing This on Purpose

The Problem

When life becomes difficult, it is easy to make assumptions about other people's intentions. When you are struggling with intense emotions and having a hard time managing, you may feel that people are purposely making things difficult or challenging for you, or deliberately testing your ability to cope. As your emotional intensity increases, so does your certainty about others' malicious intentions.

A special note about paranoia: Paranoia is the imagined or exaggerated distrust of others. It can range from distrust and suspicion on one end of the spectrum to a clinically psychotic paranoia wherein a person develops *paranoid delusions*, or false beliefs that others are out to harm, torment, or trap the person. The latter type of paranoia may require medication. In this section of this book, however, we are discussing stress-related and transient, or short-lived, episodes of paranoia.

What It Looks Like

Twenty-one-year-old Logan is having a difficult week. Her car was hit in a parking lot and the body shop is not returning her call, her friend just canceled dinner plans that were made more than a month ago, her parents are tired of hearing about her depression, and her professor, who she believes now hates her, still has not replied to her e-mail about an extension on her paper. She feels very depressed, and getting to work has been difficult. Logan begins to feel like she is doomed to fail. "It feels like no one can cut me a break." She begins to feel more anxious. She starts to wonder what she did to make everyone want to make her more depressed. Logan feels angry and hurt. "Why would people do this to me? I can't trust anyone to help me or take care of me… I hate this." Logan begins to worry about whom she can trust; she starts deleting people from her phone. She has a terrible sense of fear and loneliness.

The Practice

Here is how you address the feeling that people are doing things on purpose to upset you:

- **Notice vulnerability factors.** Ask yourself, "Given my life right now, am I more vulnerable to feeling paranoid? Am I feeling like other people are doing things on purpose to make me suffer?" If you are prone to paranoia, it is important to notice any factors that make you more vulnerable to anxiety such as physical illness, unbalanced eating, and too much or too little sleep. It is particularly important to note that drugs like cocaine, weed, and prescription stimulants can worsen paranoia. If any of these factors make you more paranoid, make a plan to address them as soon as possible. Sleep and exercise are the foundation of emotional health. While it can be easy to let these slip, addressing them will lessen the chance of becoming paranoid.

- **Use grounding.** When you become paranoid, you can have difficulty holding on to the reality of your relationships because your emotions are running very high. Paranoia can be very scary. Grounding yourself can be a helpful skill to settle your mind and decrease emotional intensity in the moment. There are many useful grounding exercises that make use of your five senses: You can use sight and notice all the things around you that are of a certain color; you can go outside and feel the fresh air on your face, or hold a piece of ice to feel cold; or you can focus on an intense taste like a sour or spicy candy. Grounding exercises can help anchor your mind when you find it spinning or when you notice paranoia.

- **Review your relationships.** It can be painful when you believe people are intentionally making your life more difficult than it already is. Your emotions can trick you into believing that people who care about you may be causing you harm. When you notice these thoughts it can be helpful to review your relationships. Ask yourself, "Would it be consistent with this person's values to want me to suffer? How has this person been supportive and helped me in the past?" Remember to always review your relationships after you have practiced grounding.

- **Challenge your assumptions.** Noticing and challenging your assumptions can help you suffer less. The thoughts that people are doing things on purpose to make you suffer are causing you suffering. Unless a person has a history of causing you harm, it is helpful to assume that he has a neutral or positive intention. A powerful way to reduce your suffering and paranoia is to practice believing that we all have good intentions and do not intentionally make others suffer. Stay away from assumptions, and be mindful of whether your own emotions are causing you to make negative assumptions or interpretations of other people's behaviors.

Checklist

☐   Have you identified vulnerability factors?

☐   Have you practiced grounding?

☐   Have you challenged your assumptions?

48 · Feeling Like Others Are Out to Get You

The Problem

You feel that others in your life are ganging up on you. You might have specific ideas about why this is happening, such as because they are getting together in order to deal with you, or you may just have a nagging suspicion without a clear idea as to why they are behaving the way that you suspect they are behaving.

What It Looks Like

Fernando is a twenty-four-year-old who has been working at a dog kennel for the past few years. He has BPD and is quite sensitive. Dog owners love him, and he gets glowing reviews from customers. Generally he gets along very well with his coworkers. In recent weeks business has been slow. The owner of the kennel has assured everyone that they will keep their jobs, but Fernando feels that he is going to get fired and that his coworkers are out to get him. He imagines being called into the office in order to be let go. He is extremely aware of what is going on around him, and he is constantly scanning his work environment for evidence that others are ganging up on him. Every time any two coworkers are talking together, Fernando is certain that their conversation is about him and that they're conspiring to find ways to get him to screw up. He also has the sense that his coworkers are looking at him, judging him negatively, and thinking that he is a screwup who should be fired.

The Practice

Here is how you address the feeling that others are out to get you:

- **Notice vulnerability factors.** Do the paranoid thoughts worsen at night when you are tired? If so, make sure that you are getting to bed early and getting a good night's sleep. Staying up late worrying about things is not going to solve the problem of paranoia. Are you using mind-altering drugs, like marijuana, that make you even more paranoid? If so, you have to be honest with yourself; even if the marijuana is providing a subjective benefit, it is not going to lessen your paranoia. Has your paranoia gone up in the context of a specific stressful situation? If so, remind yourself that you did not think that others were out to get you until the stressful situation appeared, and that responding to the paranoid feelings will not help with the stress.

- **Ask your friends.** Before jumping to the conclusion that others are out to get you, seek help from close and trusted others, like family or non-work-related friends. Review your thought process with them. Long-term trusted friends are likely to give you the most honest opinion.

- **Decide if it is a chronic or recent problem.** If the feeling that others are out to get you arose from a fairly recent situation, say within the last couple of months, it is unlikely that this is a chronic problem. This is important to note, because even though you need to deal with the situation, acute or short-term events tend to pass—and with the passing goes the paranoia as well. If you have been experiencing paranoid feelings for more than six months or so, it might be a sign of a condition that could require medication for psychosis.

- **Practice positive thinking.** Even if you are having negative thoughts, begin a practice of having a positive thought for every negative one. For instance, instead of simply saying or thinking, "They are plotting around the water-cooler about how to get rid of me," Fernando could counter that impulse with the practice of saying, "Okay, I just had a negative thought…so I have to come up with a positive or at least neutral one. Let's see… They are at the watercooler drinking because they are thirsty, and their conversation has nothing to do with me. I have no evidence whatsoever that their conversation is about me." If you regularly practice positive thinking, eventually it will become a habit.

- **Address your insecurities and lack of self-confidence.** A large part of paranoia comes from not feeling capable or good enough. Often it is not that you are paranoid per se, but that you feel "less than" others. And when you have feelings of not being good enough as your baseline emotional context, it can give rise to feelings that others are conspiring against you. So in order to address the paranoia, you must first address those insecurities. A lot of this, in turn, has to do with being confident in your capabilities. When you're confident in your abilities, you are less likely to imagine that other people are speaking badly of you or that they are out to get you. For instance, Fernando had done a wonderful job for years at the kennel. It makes no sense that the owner would let go of one of his best workers. Fernando needs to remind himself that he is great at what he does and then practice telling himself that over and over again—because it is the truth.

Checklist

☐ Have you identified vulnerability factors?

☐ Have you asked your friends?

☐ Have you determined whether it is a chronic or more recent problem?

☐ Are you practicing positive thinking?

☐ Are you addressing low self-esteem and insecurity?

CHAPTER 14

Invalidating Yourself

49 · BELIEVING THAT YOU SHOULD NOT FEEL THIS WAY

The Problem

You are feeling a strong emotion, such as anger, and then you get angry that you are feeling angry, and then you tell yourself that you should not feel angry. Telling yourself that you should not feel a certain way is often the beginning of a dangerous self-invalidating mental spiral that can quickly lead to misery.

What It Looks Like

Thirty-nine-year-old Mariya just received a promotion at work and was congratulated by her coworkers all day. As she drove home, she noticed a sense of pride in her accomplishment. However, as she approached her house her thoughts shifted. She begins wondering if she really deserves this promotion. She has screwed up so many things in her life. In fact, she is only at the job because she had to drop out of grad school. She starts to think about all the mistakes and careless errors she has made, especially in times when she was irritated or frustrated with her job or coworkers. She feels selfish for feeling a sense of pride about an accomplishment, and she feels she doesn't deserve the promotion. She starts thinking about what a failure she is and wonders if she should have turned down the promotion. Mariya keeps returning to how selfish she was all day for feeling proud of herself and happy to be recognized. She contemplates not going to work the next day.

The Practice

Here is how you address this type of self-invalidation:

- **Notice self-invalidating clues.** You must learn to identify self-invalidating thoughts—telling yourself you should not feel your emotion—in order to stop them. Here are some common *self-invalidating statements*:

  I should not feel this way.

  I am making a big deal out of nothing.

  I should just let it go.

  I am being dramatic.

  It's not that big of a deal.

  I am being stupid.

  Spend some time thinking about ways that you self-invalidate. What phrases do you use? What is the tone of your self-talk? Take notice of these details so that those phrases become part of your mindful practice of noticing. When you notice an unhelpful thought creeping up, pause and label it: "self-invalidating thought." Just noticing is the first step that will help you break the chain of this type of thinking.

- **Identify the emotion.** Once you have noticed and labeled self-invalidating thoughts, you need to identify the emotion. State the emotion explicitly in your mind. For Mariya, her emotion was pride and joy. During this practice, your mind may begin generating more self-invalidating thoughts; when this happens, return to simply labeling the emotion. Do not let your mind push you to move back into judgments or editorial statements; just stick with the emotion. Mariya might say to herself, "I am feeling proud and joyful."

- **Assess the facts.** Ask yourself, "Does this emotion fit the situation or make sense?" and "Would it be okay if my friend felt this way?" These questions will help you determine if your emotion is justified and fits the current situation. Remember: focus on the emotion, not the intensity or the situation. Stick to the facts. Make an honest assessment of the situation, and don't get caught up in self-judgments. For Mariya, pride and joy fits with getting a promotion, and she would say that it would make sense that if her friend had gotten a promotion she would feel the same way.

- **Commit to validating your emotion.** Validating your emotions is a choice and one that will decrease your suffering. Once you have noticed the invalidating thoughts, identified your emotion, and asked yourself if the emotion fits the situation, you must make a commitment to stick with self-validating. It is an active process that you will have to do over and over again, often for the same situation. If you have a long history of self-invalidation, self-validation won't come easily until you practice validating yourself a lot. When you begin to question your experience, go back to asking yourself the two questions. Then tell yourself that your emotion is valid and fits the situation. Here are some common *self-validating statements:*

It makes sense that I feel _____*.*

Other people who might have experienced this would also feel this way.

Given my past, it makes sense that I feel this way.

It is important to find words that feel authentic and honest to you. You can try using some of these statements or come up with your own.

- **Notice the impact.** Once you have self-validated, pay attention to how you feel and what is happening in your mind. Self-validating often slows down your thoughts and helps you more effectively look at or think through a situation. It also helps you not make your problem worse. If this is a new practice, at first it may feel uncomfortable. Stick with it—the impact can be profound.

Checklist

☐ Do you know the ways you self-invalidate?

☐ Have you identified the emotion that needs to be validated?

☐ Have you asked yourself what about your experience makes sense?

The Problem

You feel that you never get breaks and that things never go your way. You feel that life is unfair to you and that other people get the things that they want. The injustice of your situation feels so painful that it is almost unbearable. You may even notice powerful urges for revenge in certain situations.

What It Looks Like

When Frederick, a thirty-year-old schoolteacher, was passed over for a promotion, he complained to his spouse that life was unfair. He feels that he is always overlooked. Frederick believes that the person who got the promotion was less deserving than he was. Out of anger, Frederick posts to a social media site an unflattering photograph of his boss drinking at a colleague's wedding—a photograph that might easily be interpreted as implying that his boss has an alcohol problem.

The Practice

Life is full of injustice. You only need to turn on the TV to see war, crime, and poverty. However, when you are focused on what is unfair in your own life, it can be difficult to put your situation in perspective. Seeing yourself as a victim and believing that this is your destiny will make it difficult to see that you don't have to be life's doormat.

Here is how you address feeling that life is unfair—and avoiding engaging in revenge behavior.

- **Stop ruminating.** Ruminating on how unfair a situation is will not change it. In fact, rumination drains your energy, intensifies negative emotions, and keeps the focus on the problem rather than the solution. Continuing to think about the unfairness of a situation is not productive. Being aware of feelings and thoughts of injustice and your response to them is the first step. Next, notice if you are blaming others or repeating the thought "This is unfair." Then counter the thought with a statement like "This thought isn't helping me. The situation is what it is. I have to either accept it or try to change it."

- **Notice your urge and consider your response.** When you feel that you have been cheated and react emotionally, such as by practicing revenge, you will tend to rationalize your behavior. In Frederick's case, he admitted, "Maybe I shouldn't have posted that photo of my boss, but he deserved it!" His posting felt justified, but the long-term consequence will likely be something that he will regret.

  By noticing your urge and deciding before you act, you might realize that you are making a big deal out of a relatively small situation. For instance, recognize that it is not such a big deal when someone cuts the line when you are waiting to buy movie tickets. It may be annoying, but is it worth making a huge scene and turning what you hoped would be a pleasant night out into an evening filled with complaints of how unfair life is? Even in situations where there is a strong need to fight for justice, taking some time to plan a measured response is much more likely to lead to an effective solution than acting impulsively without thought.

- **Decide what is in your control, then act.** You can't change a past mistreatment. You can only address something that is happening in the present moment. Also, you can't easily change someone else's behavior if she isn't willing to change. You can, however, change *how* you respond to the situation. If there is an aspect of the situation that is not in your control, then you have to accept that there is nothing that you can do about it. If you missed a flight because of traffic to the airport, you cannot control that situation. This is a situation that you have to accept. What you can control is your ability to go to the ticket counter and ask for help getting onto another flight. Certainly, angrily arguing with the ticket agent about your missed flight and the unfairness of the situation is not going to make your situation any better.

Checklist

☐ Are you catching your ruminations?

☐ What is your action urge telling you to do?

☐ Do you know what you can control and what you have to accept?

51 · THINKING THAT THINGS ARE EASIER FOR OTHER PEOPLE

The Problem

All your friends are getting summer jobs while you are struggling making calls to possible summer internships. It seems so easy for them to get jobs. You are beating yourself up because you feel that you should be able to make the calls just like all your friends have done. In fact, this seems to be a pattern in your life: you always notice that it seems easy for others to do things but nearly impossible for you.

What It Looks Like

Brandon is a sixteen-year-old with BPD who has just completed his sophomore year of high school. All his friends have summer jobs, but he has been unable to find one despite being a hardworking student. The problem is that he is terrified of making phone calls to set up an interview for a prospective job. He says, "All my friends are able to call. This should be easy to do."

The Practice

The fact is, things that are easy for other people might be difficult for you, and things that are easy for you may be difficult for other people.

Here is what you can do when faced with a task that's difficult for you but seemingly easy for others:

- **Validate.** The first thing to do is to validate that the task at hand is difficult for you. In other words, determine if—given your neurobiology and your life experiences—it makes sense that the task at hand would be difficult. You are not choosing to make things difficult.

- **Identify long-term goals.** Next, determine whether what you need to do is in line with your long-term goals. For instance, in Brandon's case, getting a summer job is necessary for obtaining some summer money and job experience.

- **Identify the emotion.** Then determine the emotion that is preventing you from doing what you need to do. If you are feeling afraid, resolve to act opposite to the fear. For instance, Brandon would identify his fear of making phone calls. He would realize that the fear is preventing him from getting a job. He would then act opposite to his fear urge by making the calls.

- **Ask for help.** Perhaps the most important step of all is to ask for help. Reach out to people you trust and who understand your situation. For Brandon, this does not mean asking friends for a summer job but instead asking for help in dealing with the fear of making calls. He could ask his parents or friends to role-play a mock interview, then he would practice doing these over and over again until the task gets a little easier.

- **Throw yourself into the task.** Having validated that things are not always easy for you and practiced doing the task at hand, the final step is to face the challenge by throwing yourself fully into doing the difficult assignment.

Checklist

 Have you validated your difficulty?

 Have you determined what emotion is making it difficult to face your task?

 Have you asked for help from people you trust?

52 · Feeling Like You Are Not Normal

The Problem

You have the feeling that you are not normal. For you it is not just a matter of comparing yourself to other people, it's the sense that there is something fundamentally wrong with your brain.

What It Looks Like

Kristin is twenty years old and feels that there is something fundamentally wrong with who she is. She does not see others' sense of humor, can't understand why others can be calm when she is so outraged by injustice, and gets frustrated when others don't see how different she is. Kristin does not judge others' behavior. She accepts that others are normal. She feels that her struggles are simply a reflection of how *not* normal she is. She equates her abnormality to a physical abnormality—one in her brain. "If I were eight feet tall," Kristin explains, "I would not be normal, but at least people would know that because they can see it. With my brain, people just can't see it, so they don't get it. It makes me suffer. If I had a different brain then I would be normal."

The Practice

Normal behavior and thinking is subjective and often only recognized in contrast to what is considered abnormal. Typically, normality is seen as good and desirable, while abnormality is often judged as bad or undesirable. But what's opposite of normal is not necessarily abnormal—it can simply be different. For instance, the opposite of a carnivore is an herbivore. One might consider carnivore normal, but that is not to say that an herbivore is abnormal.

Here is how you can begin to change your thinking about not being normal:

- **Categorize "not normal" as a judgment.** It is true that you may perceive things very differently from other people and that you may struggle with the sense that your brain is distorting experiences. You are who you are and have the brain that you have. One response is to say you are "not normal" and accept this. Quite another is to harshly judge yourself as "not normal" in a way that causes suffering. It is possible that your thinking is not always clear. If you have daily distortions of reality with the clinical symptoms of delusions and hallucinations, there may be medications that can help; however, if your thoughts are simply ones that don't resonate with the people around you, and your thoughts don't cause you to suffer, then likely your thinking is simply different.

- **Define what you mean by "not normal."** Most of your experiences in life will be typical, so when you say you are "not normal," be clear. Typically what people with BPD mean when they say that they are not normal is that they have the kinds of thoughts and emotions that keep them miserable while others don't seem to suffer as intensely, if at all. Rather than say, "I am a terrible, horrible person… I'm not normal," be specific to your situation, such as saying, "All my friends like rap music but I like country, and I feel that my taste in music is not normal." By describing the experience that makes you conclude you are not normal, you can tackle that specific thought.

- **Practice accepting yourself.** Just because someone doesn't agree with what you are doing, how you are feeling, or how you are behaving doesn't mean you are not normal or that you need to change. You are who you are even when others disagree or don't understand your experiences. Practice saying, "This is who I am, and I accept myself." The more you can accept yourself, the more others will too.

- **Self-compassion changes everything.** Judging yourself as abnormal is not helpful. Even more than practicing accepting yourself, practice self-compassion and love for yourself. Say to yourself, "This is who I am, and I can love myself."

Checklist

☐ Have you recognized that calling yourself "not normal" is a judgment?

☐ Have you specifically defined what you mean by "not normal"?

☐ Have you accepted yourself?

☐ What acts of self-compassion have you done?

53 · FEELING LIKE YOU CAN'T TRUST YOUR DECISIONS

The Problem

You have an important decision to make, but you are sitting on the fence. You feel afraid to make a choice because you are worried that you will make the wrong decision. And then, when your intuition tells you that one choice is better than the other, you don't trust it—even when you know what is best for you.

What It Looks Like

When twenty-two-year-old Eleanor had to decide whether to switch majors in college, she was stuck. On the one hand, she had devoted three years of her life studying business; however, in the past year she had taken a psychology elective and found her psychology classes to be much more interesting than her business classes. She worried that if she switched majors she would disappoint her father, a business-man, and that she would have wasted some of her college years. She could not decide what to do. She began to question everything, asking herself things like "If I can't decide about this, how will I ever be able to decide about anything? Even if I did switch, how do I know I won't switch again? If I switch, will I be successful? It's a given that I can always go and work for my father; will I be able to get a job as a psychologist?" Every night she goes to bed hoping that she will know what to do the next day, only to find that she is stuck asking herself the same questions, having the same doubts, unable to trust in her own decisions.

The Practice

When you are stuck with an important decision to make, here are some steps to help you learn to trust your own wisdom:

- **Make a list of pros and cons.** Write down the positives and negatives of decision A, and create a similar list for decision B. Then decide which items on the list are consistent with your long-term goals and weigh those as more important. Let's say that there are many more pros with decision B than the pros of decision A; however, if the pros in decision A are more in keeping with your life goals, then go with A. For instance, Eleanor has "Happiness and fulfillment" in her pros of a psychology major; she has "money, Dad's approval, nearly completed course, future job being set, and less of a hassle to switch" for continuing with a business major. In her case, happiness and fulfillment are more important than the many reasons for continuing in business, because they work toward her long-term goals.

- **Avoid people who undermine your self-confidence.** One of Eleanor's suite-mates has a habit of giving people advice whether they want it or not. She repeatedly tells Eleanor that she is too indecisive to become a good psychologist, along with other unhelpful things. Instead of people like Eleanor's suite-mate, seek out people who are curious and prepared to understand what you are going through.

- **Make a commitment and stick to it.** Self-trust is a skill that has to and can be practiced. The best way to start is to make small daily and then weekly commitments—and stick to them. For instance, you might commit to go to bed earlier every night for a week. Or pledge to read a book rather than watch TV, or to go to the gym rather than eat a bag of chips. These may seem like trivial choices to make, but the idea is that you are practicing making one decision over another.

- **Be kind to yourself.** Don't beat yourself up for being unable to decide what to do. Or if you are judging yourself, notice that you are doing so. Are you beating yourself up because you have done something that crosses your values, or is it the "voice" of someone else in your life that you perceive is judging you? For instance, in Eleanor's case, she imagined her father telling her that she was ungrateful and indecisive. She imagined her father telling her she was not good enough. Rather than automatically judging yourself the way that you imagine others would judge you, practice being more understanding toward yourself by saying something like "It makes sense that you have this dilemma. Let's see what I can do to figure this out."

- **Listen to your own wisdom.** When people don't trust themselves, they normally seek guidance from everyone else. It's okay to ask for help from people you trust, but don't let others' considerations be the ultimate factor. They may have different perspectives on the decision you need to make; weigh them, then ask yourself, "What do my own intuition and wisdom tell me to do?"

Checklist

- ☐ Have you made a list of pros and cons of each choice?
- ☐ Are you being kind to yourself?
- ☐ Are you listening to your inner wisdom?

Epilogue

Dear Reader,

Borderline personality disorder is not a lifelong condition, and the majority of people with BPD will not live lives of unremitting suffering. Your life will get better. These are not simply some reassuring words but a statement of fact supported by research studies that have followed people with BPD for more than twenty years.

However, until recovery sets in, the symptoms of BPD can lead to suffering. So with this book we set out to give you some ideas that we hope you will find helpful when dealing with typical challenges. The skills we've shared will allow you to interact with your emotions and with other people in a more effective way. This is a coaching guide that you can continue to reference, one that you can keep on your bedside table, read on the bus on your way to school, or keep in a drawer at work to look at whenever you need some inspiration.

If the ideas in this book are new to you, then, as with any new learning practice, repetition is essential in acquiring the skills that will see you through difficult moments. Or perhaps the techniques provide a different perspective on skills you already know. Either way, as with all learning, the more you practice these new, effective ways of coping, the better you will be at using them, and the more these new ways of managing your life and emotions will become a part of your natural reactions. If you have taken these exercises seriously, you are already well on your way. Remember to continue to practice. You *will* become more effective.

We have dedicated our professional lives to the treatment of BPD. And we will continue to do so. We share many interesting ideas and research in real time on our Twitter accounts, @blaisemd and @GillianPsyD. We hope you will follow us.

As you continue on your path to healing we wish you a skillful journey. And if this book is a part of it, we are happy to have been a part of your life along the way.

Sincerely,

Blaise and Gillian

References

Bushman, B. J. 2002. "Does Venting Anger Feed or Extinguish the Flame? Catharsis, Rumination, Distraction, Anger, and Aggressive Responding." *Personality and Social Psychology Bulletin* 28(6): 724–31.

Fierce Inc. 2013. "Toxic Employees: Colleagues Advocate Confrontation, While Companies Perceived as Too Tolerant: Coworker Negativity 'Extremely Debilitating' to Team Morale According to 78 Percent of Employees." September 19. http://www.fierceinc.com/uploads/Press Release-Infographics/ToxicEmployeesFinalRelease.pdf.

Grant, B. F., S. P. Chou, R. B. Goldstein, et al. 2008. "Prevalence, Correlates, Disability, and Comorbidity of *DSM-IV* Borderline Personality Disorder: Results from the Wave 2 National Epidemiologic Survey on Alcohol and Related Conditions." *Journal of Clinical Psychiatry* 69 (4): 533–45.

Linehan, M. M. 1993a. *Cognitive Behavioral Treatment of Borderline Personality Disorder.* New York: Guilford Press.

Linehan, M. M. 1993b. *Skills Training Manual for Treating Borderline Personality Disorder.* New York: Guilford Press.

Linehan, M. M. 2014a. *DBT® Skills Training Handouts and Worksheets.* Second Edition, New York: Guilford Press.

Linehan, M. M. 2014b. *DBT® Skills Training Manual.* Second Edition, New York: Guilford Press.

Snyder, M. 1974. "Self-monitoring of Expressive Behavior." *Journal of Personality and Social Psychology* 30: 526–37.

Blaise Aguirre, MD, is assistant professor of psychiatry at Harvard Medical School, and an expert in child, adolescent, and adult psychotherapy, including dialectical behavior therapy (DBT), and medication evaluation and management. He is founding medical director of McLean 3East—a unique residential DBT program for young women exhibiting self-endangering behaviors and borderline personality disorder (BPD) traits. Dr. Aguirre has been a staff psychiatrist at McLean since 2000, and is internationally recognized for his extensive work in the treatment of mood and personality disorders in adolescents. He lectures regularly in Europe, Africa, and the Middle East on DBT and BPD. Dr. Aguirre is author of *Borderline Personality Disorder in Adolescents* and *Depression (Biographies of Disease)*, and coauthor of *Mindfulness for Borderline Personality Disorder* and *Helping Your Troubled Teen*.

Gillian Galen, PsyD, is instructor of psychology at Harvard Medical School. She is program director and assistant director of training for the 3East Intensive Residential Program at the Harvard-affiliated McLean Hospital—a unique residential dialectical behavior therapy (DBT) program for young women exhibiting self-endangering behaviors and borderline personality disorder (BPD) traits. She specializes in adolescent psychotherapy, including DBT. She has a particular interest in using mindfulness and yoga in the treatment of BPD and other psychiatric illnesses. Galen has been a registered yoga instructor since 2008. She is coauthor of *Mindfulness for Borderline Personality Disorder*.

Foreword author **Alec Miller, PsyD**, is cofounder of Cognitive and Behavioral Consultants of Westchester, LLP, in White Plains, NY. He is professor of clinical psychiatry and behavioral sciences, chief of child and adolescent psychology, director of the Adolescent Depression and Suicide Program, and director of clinical services at PS 8 School-Based Mental Health Program. Miller has become internationally known in the areas of adolescent depression and suicidology, non-suicidal self-injury, borderline personality disorder (BPD), and dialectical behavior therapy (DBT). He has authored numerous articles and book chapters, and is coauthor of *Dialectical Behavior Therapy with Suicidal Adolescents* and *Childhood Maltreatment*.

FROM OUR PUBLISHER—

As the publisher at New Harbinger and a clinical psychologist since 1978, I know that emotional problems are best helped with evidence-based therapies. These are the treatments derived from scientific research (randomized controlled trials) that show what works. Whether these treatments are delivered by trained clinicians or found in a self-help book, they are designed to provide you with proven strategies to overcome your problem.

Therapies that aren't evidence-based—whether offered by clinicians or in books—are much less likely to help. In fact, therapies that aren't guided by science may not help you at all. That's why this New Harbinger book is based on scientific evidence that the treatment can relieve emotional pain.

This is important: if this book isn't enough, and you need the help of a skilled therapist, use the following resources to find a clinician trained in the evidence-based protocols appropriate for your problem. And if you need more support—a community that understands what you're going through and can show you ways to cope—resources for that are provided below, as well.

Real help is available for the problems you have been struggling with. The skills you can learn from evidence-based therapies will change your life.

Matthew McKay, PhD
Publisher, New Harbinger Publications

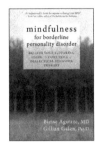
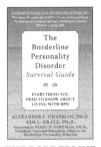
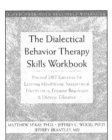
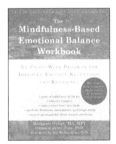
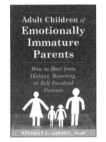
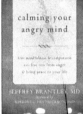
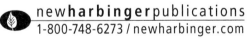 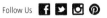

Real change *is* possible

For more than forty-five years, New Harbinger has published proven-effective self-help books and pioneering workbooks to help readers of all ages and backgrounds improve mental health and well-being, and achieve lasting personal growth. In addition, our spirituality books offer profound guidance for deepening awareness and cultivating healing, self-discovery, and fulfillment.

Founded by psychologist Matthew McKay and Patrick Fanning, New Harbinger is proud to be an independent, employee-owned company. Our books reflect our core values of integrity, innovation, commitment, sustainability, compassion, and trust. Written by leaders in the field and recommended by therapists worldwide, New Harbinger books are practical, accessible, and provide real tools for real change.

newharbingerpublications